COMMON SENSE
IN THERAPY

A Handbook for the
Mental Health Worker

Common Sense in Therapy

A HANDBOOK FOR THE MENTAL HEALTH WORKER

by
Yoosuf A. Haveliwala, M.D.
Albert E. Scheflen, M.D.
and
Norman Ashcraft, Ph.D.

BRUNNER/MAZEL, *Publishers* • New York

Library of Congress Cataloging in Publication Data

Haveliwala, Yoosuf A.   1934-
  Common sense in therapy.
  1. Psychotherapy.   I. Scheflen, Albert E., joint author.   II. Ashcraft, Norman, 1936-   joint author.   III. Title.

RC480.H37   616.8'914   79-13340
ISBN 0-87630-203-7

Published by
BRUNNER/MAZEL, INC.
19 Union Square, New York, New York 10003

MANUFACTURED IN THE UNITED STATES OF AMERICA

Preface

We wrote this book because we felt there was a gap in the existing literature. There are any number of books in the field of mental health that speak to the professional though they usually are weighted in an academic direction or written from the perspective of a particular doctrine. There are also books written for the paraprofessional.

What appeared to be lacking was an intermediate view that dealt with the several procedures and styles of modern mental health and yet was also addressed to the front-line workers who do mental health on a daily basis. This book is written for that audience and especially for the beginning worker, that person who is just starting out in a career in mental health.

We have made an attempt to stay with practical issues, to picture mental health as the worker must. At the same time, we felt such a handbook should also include a brief survey of some of the major ideas of the field. We do not think a mental health worker should be limited to knowing only one doctrine, or one approach, or a couple of convenient techniques. Yet far too much of our education stresses one principle over the others. This handbook attempts to expose the reader to several approaches, although it does not fully explore every major method or technique.

In the background lies the core principle of this book: *Practicing mental health involves staying human and using common sense.* Sometimes this means working *with* a client and sometimes this means appreciating one's place in the total organization in which one works.

The book is divided into three parts. The first part deals with defining the problem and assessing the situation. Part II explores the selection of a therapy and provides a view of various methods and techniques. Part III addresses the place of the worker within the system of mental health. Mental health workers do not offer help to clients in a vacuum. We must have a place to work and we do our work within a particular organizational setting. Understanding how organizations are structured helps us to use the system for our own benefit and for the benefit of our clients.

Acknowledgments

We owe a great deal to many people who have contributed in various ways to the making of this book. All our friends and colleagues at the Harlem Valley Psychiatric Center deserve our gratitude.

We would especially like to thank Ronald Gatsik and Marilyn Oswald of Harlem Valley Psychiatric Center, Kitty LaPerriere of The Ackerman Institute, and Elaine Pasquali of the School of Nursing, Adelphi University, for reading portions of early drafts and for their useful comments and advice. We would also like to call attention to the help offered by the staff of the Sound Shore Clinic with Dr. Jane Ferber as Chief of Service. However, the authors remain solely responsible for the content of the book.

Finally, our thanks to Louise Hubbard for guiding parts of the manuscript through the details of typing and duplicating and to Nancy Paolucci and Christine Schopen for typing portions of the manuscript.

Contents

Introduction

This is a handbook for people working with people. It is written as an aid primarily for front-line mental health professionals, that is, for those workers who must make decisions on the spot, those workers who must take action with clients, those workers who *do* mental health.

Our goal is not to offer another ponderous textbook. But neither do we wish to offer formulas for shortcuts that oversimplify and distort the knowledge learned in mental health.

A handbook is meant to be a guide. It cannot substitute for actual experience in working with clients and it cannot replace knowledge of the various technical concepts that help define modern mental health. A guide can, however, be a help in everyday practice.

Everyone has favorite guiding principles that serve as a backdrop for daily decisions. We offer the following three because they provide a brief but practical summary of the ideas underlining this handbook.

Doing mental health is:

1. *Using comomn sense.*
2. *Doing with the client, not at him.*
3. *Using the resources available to you.*

Doing Mental Health Is Using Common Sense

One of us once answered a client who asked, "How does your professional background prepare you to help us?" with "I see myself as an expert trained in common sense."

Using common sense in the helping situation means using the common knowledge open to anyone who has become an adult member of this society. This knowledge is the knowledge that has been tested and found practical. Applying common experience in therapy means remembering to be practical and not letting a cherished professional doctrine or method become a dogmatic explanation for behavior and events. We should not fall into the trap of believing that a tactic can be applied to all situations. Tactics are useful only when we use common sense to guide us in their use.

Let your common sense guide your choice of words. Technical language may be convenient for the helper, but it probably does not help the client. Words and concepts that have become second nature to us can be misunderstood or not understood by the one asking for help. Besides, a mental health worker's tendency to speak in jargon may simply reflect the need to have a crutch at that moment. On the other hand, it is not necessary to go to the other extreme. We need not resort to cliché and folksy chitchat in order to do jargon-free therapy.

Avoiding locking yourself into a static treatment plan. Classifications are always unsatisfactory when put into day-to-day use. Situations are relative, responding not only to the demands of the personal problems of the moment, but also to rules, laws and policies, as well as to available resources.

Situations flow through a process. A frozen therapeutic approach ignores the dynamics of the various problems of daily living. Doing mental health is like a journey in which each step includes a series of gates. The gate we choose opens certain pathways and temporarily closes others. Each pathway leads to another set of gates. The more flexible we are in our decisions, the more manageable this system of pathways becomes for the client.

In using common sense, we learn to appreciate the meaning of feelings. The anthropologist, Edmund Carpenter, tells the story that after having spent many years living and working in the far north, he was asked by an Eskimo woman one day, "Do we smell and is it offensive to you?" He did not attempt to mask his feelings nor hide the truth. He answered her in the affirmative. The woman responded, for she seemed relieved to learn the truth. She added, "You smell and it's

offensive to us. We wondered if we smelled and if it offended you."
A new element of attachment was born in that exchange, an element
made possible through sharing. They came to appreciate the human
quality in each of them.

We should treat our feelings practically by putting them to work.
Feelings cannot be divorced from social intercourse, and therapy is a
form of social intercourse. If we believe we can always mask our feelings and attitudes, we kid only ourselves. We must decide as we go
along how much of our own feelings and thoughts we will reveal to
those around us, and how and when we will encourage our clients to
reveal theirs.

In theory we may believe we can work with any client. In practice
we come to recognize early that it is almost impossible to work with
a client we dislike. We might be able to turn that dislike into a thera-
peutically tactical situation, but we might also find it advisable to break
off the relationship. All too often therapists labor on with a client to
no one's practical advantage. We should not be afraid to end relationships. *Sometimes the best treatment is for us not to be the one treating
that person.*

Doing Mental Health Is Doing with the Client, Not at Him

As we engage in the daily task of trying to understand people who
are asking for help, we must learn to appreciate the quality of that
asking and to respond in kind. *If we are ready to help, we should be
ready to see, listen and appreciate.*

An important ingredient here is communication. In the academic
sense of helping, we can sit and listen and offer our interpretations or
advice. Yet, this cannot be enough. It is especially not enough in the
busy clinic that is the setting for much of today's mental health care.
We ask you to reach back to the root of the word communicate—*to
share together.* We must learn to do more than exchange views; we
must get in *with* the client.

While training to become mental health workers, we have heard
those arguments that stress the value of establishing "rapport." Rapport is valuable, but not enough. We argue for the idea of *appreciating.*
We must sense the client's mood and style of asking for help, while

merging our ideas of the present situation with those of the client. This means giving validity to the client's remarks and interpretations, as well as to our own. In helping we become part of the situation. The sense of detachment is fine in theory. On the front line we soon learn how involved we become. *Being aware of that participation helps us keep on top of it, helps us maintain control, and helps us be ever mindful of working with the person.*

Doing Mental Health Is Using the Resources Available to You

Doing mental health often involves sitting in a relatively private room doing psychotherapy or case management with just two people present, you and the client. How did the two of you come to be there?

The answer seems simple enough. You have a job as a mental health worker. You have made this career choice and you have prepared yourself for this job. The client suffers from some problem that has eventually resulted in his being here. He probably has been referred to your service by some other agency, family member, or friend. But whether he has gone through one gate in the mental health world or several, he is now alone with you.

This is how the two of you got there. But should you be there together? Is this client suitable for the service you have to offer? Is there a danger present and can you handle it? Should there be more than two of you present?

Perhaps the two of you are ill-matched. Your responsibility at this point is not to kid yourself. Seek advice, a consultation or co-therapist, and remember, the best therapy *you* can offer may well be referring this client to another therapist.

Perhaps the service you have to offer is not suitable for the client at this moment. The most pressing problem may not be the need for psychotherapy, but the need for medical assistance. Perhaps the client is a danger to himself or to others and the resources of hospitalization seem in order. Whatever the case, it is your responsibility *to make an evaluation of the client's* needs of the moment. If medical attention is called for, then see to that need and make another appointment for the two of you to get together at an appropriate time in the future.

The problem may well be the result of the two of you sitting alone in the room. Maybe there is danger, or maybe there is no danger, but the situation is too hot for you to handle alone. *Make use of the therapeutic supports open to you.* You may need a consultation or a co-therapist. Maybe you need the entire family present and a co-therapist to help you deal with the complexity.

All too often our training prepares us for one-to-one therapy. But in practice, mental health increasingly involves the need for more people present. Do not hesitate to realize that you should not tackle some problems alone. No matter how broad our experience, there are crises in which we should seek help. Sometimes the issue is clear. At other times we may kid ourselves through pride or a sense of professionalism that obscures the need for assistance.

Doing mental health together is remembering that you are not alone. Make use of these support systems. If you work in a clinic there are colleagues and supervisors who are available. In turn you are available to them. If you are in private practice, advice, consultation, even referrals, are open via the telephone and, in some cases, via two-way videotape hookup.

COMMON SENSE IN THERAPY

A Handbook for the Mental Health Worker

I. What Is the Problem?

The first step in any situation involves making an initial assessment. This may mean some quick thinking if we sense the presence of an emergency. But emergencies, crises, or routine contacts all include information-taking before action-taking. If it is an emergency we need to know what kind of emergency. We need to know, too, something about available resources, for the action we take more than likely will involve mustering our own resources, as well as those of our clients. An initial assessment, then, is critical in forming the basis for action.

1. Emergencies and Crises

Mental health workers rely heavily on the development of the therapeutic alliance as a means of helping others. Yet, there are moments when this familiar process is not enough. Emergencies and crises are such instances. We are forced to take some definitive action, whether our involvement is no more than answering the telephone at the clinic, being on night duty on a ward, or being told by someone else that our client is trying desperately to reach us. Help of a special kind is being asked and that need demands an appropriate response from us.

Chapter Topics

5

1:1. Emergencies and Crises

The words emergency and crisis can have a wide range of meanings. In some uses the terms overlap and sometimes they are used synonymously. We have chosen to picture emergencies and crises as follows:

    I. Emergencies:
        A. Non-mental health emergencies
        B. Mental hospital and psychiatric emergencies
   II. Crises:
        A. The consultation or screening situation
        B. The crisis intervention or team situation
        C. The multi-client or family situation

Emergencies demand the response of others better equipped than the mental health worker. Such agencies as the police, emergency wards, or the fire department have both the resources and the expertise to handle emergencies. Mental health workers do not. We can assist a person in obtaining proper help and we can later pick up the case and thereby bring the expertise of mental health to the scene.

Threats of suicide, homicide, or other forms of violence, as well as sickness or accidents, demand action, but not that of psychotherapy. The police, courts, fire departments, ambulance, medical hospital, etc., are the appropriate institutions to meet the non-mental health emergency.

The second type of emergency in our scheme is the psychiatric emergency. At this moment, this type of situation requires resources beyond the reach of most mental health workers. Hospitalization may be repugnant to some mental health workers, but there are clearly those instances when the mental hospital is best equipped to tackle the immediate problem. Later, as the emergency is cooled down, the mental health worker can enter the scene to assist in the process of returning the individual to a healthier life-style.

Emergencies are handled by other professionals. Crises belong to the mental health worker. But we consider many crises too hot for the individual to handle alone. A colleague, supervisor, or co-therapist should be brought in to help with the immediate situation. If this path is not open, then the services of a consultant with special skills or legal backing who can help both us *and* the client should be sought. Finally, a crisis will likely involve more people than just the individual client. Mustering the client's family or network may be the most appropriate action of the moment.

1:2. The Initial Screen: The Telephone Call

The first contact with the mental health world is likely to be made via the telephone. The cry for help, the crisis call, even the emergency, frequently begin with the telephone. We might as well come to appreciate the importance of what we might label *telephone mental health,* because that is where a great deal of our professional time will be spent.

The most critical time to appreciate doing one's job over the phone occurs as we answer and the voice on the other end anxiously asks for help. These are the emergency and crisis calls. On the basis of nothing more than our experience and the electronic sound of another voice, we must make some rapid decisions.

Our best advice is to *receive the call at face value*. This is no time to make the decision that the call is a hoax. *Believe the caller* and begin to make initial assessments. Is this an emergency or a crisis? If it is an emergency, act appropriately and now; if it is a crisis, listen.

If it is a crisis, our initial assessment must learn if the problem is

acute or chronic. If acute, we must deal with it now! If chronic, we
begin to ask why this call is being made at this time. We want to
ask questions, such as can they get into the office or must we go to
them. If the caller can make an appointment to come in, even if that
means getting down to the office right away, the context for crisis resolution has already begun.

In any crisis call, be an active therapist. Do not sit back and employ
the usual psychodynamic models. Move in and get the answers to key
questions *quickly.* A quiet, cool, and concerned manner offers the
caller an immediate kind of support, a support of reassurance. The
answers will be critical in our overall assessment of the immediacy of
the issue. Our job is to *identify the here-and-now problem and deal
with that!* Later, once the crisis has been cooled down, we can develop
a more psychodynamic treatment plan.

Take action with all telephone calls. In many cases this action will
probably involve no more than making a referral, setting up an appointment, or offering some helpful advice to a client who is having
difficulty planning a weekend trip. Even if the call is not a crisis,
remember the importance of doing something. We all know how an-
noying it is to be given the runaround by bureaucrats. We are in a
helping profession, so let's help!

1:3. Who Is Calling?

"This is Miss Williams. I'm the social worker here at the City
Agency for Delinquent Children. I have a young man here ..."

"This is Mrs. Moreno. My husband is very sick. He just sits and
stares. I called our doctor who ..."

"This is Doctor Smith. There is an interesting case of anxiety neurosis in a young woman who needs psychotherapy. I simply can't take any more cases, so . . ."

"My husband is away and I don't know what to do. My daughter has locked herself in her room and I'm afraid. You see, we live on the fourteenth floor, and . . ."

Sometimes the caller does not immediately identify herself and we must ask. In these four examples we know who is calling—a social worker, a wife, a pyschiatrist, and a mother.

But there is more to the question of who is calling than merely a name or a title. We want to know right away what relation the caller has to the problem, as well as to the troubled person.

Miss Williams is a social worker. Fine. We can work from there. How well does she know this particular adolescent? Is she just passing on a name because she, too, received a telephone call, or is this young man someone whom she has worked with before?

Dr. Smith is a psychiatrist who wants us to take an "interesting case." But has he interviewed the woman and made an appraisal, or is he, too, passing on a telephone call? What leads him to his conclusions?

There are many motives for calling and we must discover them. Mrs. Moreno may have put up with her husband's behavior for 20 years, but this evening she has reached the limit. She is distraught, feels terrified and vindictive, but has no more cause for alarm today than yesterday. Knowingly, or unknowingly, she may be setting us up to hospitalize her husband.

A more insidious "who" might be Dr. Smith, who is a wealthy and prestigious psychiatrist who has a full case load. The woman he is discussing inadvertently called on him. She comes from a low-income family, with no visible means of financial support. His classification may be no more valid than the buck-passing he is attempting.

As we listen and ask questions, we begin to form a picture of the "who." We listen to the words and we attune ourselves to voice qualities, innuendoes, hesitations, cadence of the speech, hostility, anxiety in the person's voice, style of speaking, and so on.

1:4. What Is the Problem?

As soon as we have identified ourselves, the caller begins to set us up for the problem.

Mrs. Moreno claims her husband is very sick.

Dr. Smith says he has a patient with an anxiety neurosis.

"My daughter is locked in her room."

At this point, it doesn't matter if the story we are hearing is fabricated or not. We listen and make our judgments and act accordingly. But we must be aware of the process, for this awareness provides us with a broader picture of the context in which the problem will be described.

We listen to the claim: *A* person is named. *A* person has the problem. We are told that the problem is *that* person's behavior. But many of us know from experience that the identified person is rarely the problem alone. Mrs. Moreno claims that her husband is very sick, but we learn in the course of the telephone conversation that she has seen him like this many times in the course of their 20 years of marriage. What happened in their home to warrant today's call? *However,* this telephone conversation is not the moment to interrupt and challenge Mrs. Moreno. We will want to know more about the problem and especially how critical it is so that we can make our decision on how to act. This is not the appropriate moment for deciding who the patient *should be*. We must deal with the here-and-now as it is being presented.

Miss Williams, the social worker, tells us that the boy is "acting out." We know this is trade jargon for describing so-called unacceptable or unsocial behavior. We don't want classifications. We want details and more information. Diplomatically we press for a more detailed description of the problem.

Dr. Smith tells us the woman has anxiety problems. We take his remarks at face value and imagine that the woman is troubled without knowing why. In our heads we may make conjectures, attributing her panic to sexual or aggressive fantasies. But the conjectures must remain what they are. At this moment, we are unable to conduct an interview with the identified patient, so we continue to seek more details. We may be tempted also to take a detailed personal history and attempt a preliminary psychodynamic interpretation. *But this is not the time or place. On the telephone, we have other, more urgent business to attend to.*

We have practical decisions to make. What do we do first and how we do it? Is the crisis at a critical stage? Is there an immediate danger?

Possibly the daughter will not remain locked in that fourteenth floor room while we take a long history from her mother. It may be that she might use that moment to take some more drastic action. In this instance, it makes little sense to begin a psychodynamic interview. This is not the point to worry about the motivations of mother or daughter or who, in fact, should be the patient. We must take action on the basis of the urgency of the mother's call, even though we lack other important information. That information will be forthcoming as we become more assured of a calmer situation.

Our questions grow more direct: We ask Mrs. Moreno whether her husband has ever been violent? If so, how did she handle it in the past? Is he violent now? Has he threatened violence? Has he threatened suicide? *We work on the immediacy of the problem.*

At the appropriate moment we must learn the previous history of this *particular problem or symptom.* Do not seek a case history in general. Has Mr. Moreno been like this before? If so, what happened? The distraught mother who is calling from her fourteenth floor apartment has already cued us on how to assess the situation. There is the hint of violence because she said that she was afraid and she pointedly told us in the beginning that they lived on the fourteenth floor. Okay, has this happened before? Any suggestion of suicide demands that we take action. If that mother is afraid and if her daughter has threatened suicide in whatever form, this is not the moment to practice psychotherapy.

1:5. What Is the Situation?

We must learn what resources are available to deal with the problem. Can we look to others for help in managing the immediate problem? Is a home visit necessary at this time? The severity and immediacy of the problem cannot be separated from the setting as we attempt to make our assessment for action.

We have a picture of Mr. Moreno and we have concluded that he must be seen by a professional soon. Can Mrs. Moreno get her husband to the clinic? Do they have a car? Can relatives or friends help her? Is Mrs. Moreno composed and physically capable of bringing her husband to the office? Our decisions will follow from the answers to these kinds of questions.

We question Miss Williams more closely about the nature of supports and about the present state of affairs. Will the young man be willing to come to the clinic? Does he live with a responsible family? We receive affirmative answers and we also believe, given the social worker's account, that there is no immediate danger of criminal action. We proceed accordingly.

The situation is different with Dr. Smith's referral. The young woman with the "anxiety neurosis" lives alone and is quite depressed. The psychiatrist has spoken to her only on the telephone, but he thinks she has no immediate family. Until we telephone her we cannot reach a decision. But we are predisposed to suspect that we cannot count on her coming to us. A home visit may be in order.

We must not overlook the immediacy of situations like the woman and her daughter who has locked herself in a room on the fourteenth floor. Principles of assessment must yield here to the dangers of suicide. How far away is she? How long will it take us to get there? Who can help now? How about the building superintendent? How about the police? These are questions that guide emergency decisions.

Our own resources form part of the situation as well. When we answer Miss Williams', Mrs. Moreno's, or Dr. Smith's telephone call, where and how do we fit into the situation? Are we a member of a crisis team? Do we have a walk-in clinic support system which is equipped to manage a critical crisis? Do we work in a hospital where medical supports are immediately available? Or do we have a private practice with no built-in backups? Where we sit will play no small part in how we will respond to these calls and how we will shape our decisions.

1:6. The Non-Medical Emergency

A man stood on the parapet of an office building. He looked as if he might jump. A medical student happened by and volunteered to help. He went up to the roof and spoke to the man, trying out an idea he had heard in one of his lectures at the medical college. The student accused the man of trying to manipulate other people. The man jumped.

Unless we are specialists in suicide prevention, we ought to keep our particular expertise for another time and place.

There is no reason to avoid lending a helping hand, but the assistance should be offered in conjunction with getting the right kind of people to do the job. The police and firemen have equipment and some of them have a great deal of experience in dealing with people like the man standing on a ledge of the roof.

Mrs. Elliot, a social worker, agreed to see a patient one evening after the clinic was closed. She knew the patient to be paranoid and easily excited, yet she thought she could help. She sat with him in a virtually deserted building in a closed room, relying faithfully on her psychotherapeutic experience. She asked him questions about what was troubling him at this moment. The patient turned suddenly hostile, growing more excited with each passing moment. Mrs. Elliot tried to calm him down, adopting a quiet and persuasive manner, a technique she usually found practical and wise. The patient began threatening her and yelling at her. Fortunately, another colleague happened by and together the two therapists tried to deal with the patient. It soon became evident to Mrs. Elliot that matters were going from bad to worse and that no technique seemed to alter the man's violent temperament. She excused herself and called the police.

What had started as a psychotherapeutic session evolved very rapidly into an emergency. In our opinion, Mrs. Elliot acted wisely, for in preventing violence she not only prevented someone from getting hurt, but she also maintained her credibility as a therapist. Her expertise was of little value in the face of an imminent change from verbal attack to physical attack. However, we should caution Mrs. Elliot to be more circumspect in making appointments with potentially dangerous clients when she is alone at the clinic.

There is a delicate balance, for in any emergency we will be prompted to pitch in and help. But that help does not call for foolish heroics or a misplaced dedication to go it alone no matter what. *Doing something is not the same as doing everything.*

1:7. The Medical Emergency

"Mrs. Jones is lying on the couch unconscious," the caller tells us. "What should I do? She's a patient at your clinic and there is a half empty bottle of sleeping pills on the floor."

We don't need any more information. Mrs. Jones needs medical attention. We are faced with an immediate decision. Should we trust the person to call an ambulance or should we make that call? The answer may well rest with our feeling for the situation. *The critical point is to see that realistic action is taken.* We can ask the person to telephone for an ambulance and then we may notify the police, just as a precaution. Or we may take matters more directly into our own hands.

Not all situations present themselves as emergencies. We are sitting with Mr. and Mrs. Smith completing a rather long psychiatric history. Mr. Smith is dull, lethargic, and inattentive. His wife does most of the talking. Mr. Smith's inattention doesn't catch our concern until we pick up a comment of Mrs. Smith. Her husband is a diabetic. Altered states of consciousness should key us to ask about diabetes.

Headaches can be a warning too. They can be a reaction to the psychotherapeutic process, or stress, tension, or what not. But a severe, persisting headache with accompanying visual symptoms and impaired consciousness could also indicate a brain tumor, a brain hemorrhage or severe hypertension. Don't take the risk. Get a medical consultation or insist on a medical clearance before making an appointment.

General weakness, fatigue and an inability to eat are characteristic in psychogenic problems and stress, but the symptoms also may indicate anemia, an early cancer, or a host of other physical problems.

Anxiety is often accompanied by blurred vision. Patients on the phenothiazines commonly experience this symptom as well. But when there is clear double vision, when the patient sees two distinct images, medical advice is in order.

In all cases where we suspect a serious medical problem, we should consider the possibility of a medical emergency.

1:8. The Acute Psychosis

A relative tells us that someone is acting strangely or is uncustomarily belligerent and abusive. Or we hear that Tom has disappeared without a word, or Mary has run out of the house screaming. The person is pacing about, not eating, sitting with a fixed stare, and so on. The troubled individual is not clear about who he is or what he is perceiving. Other people seem strange to him. Perhaps he sees visions or hears voices.

But the mental health worker does not have to be told in detail about the manifestations of psychosis. If the description of the patient suggests psychosis, we must try to determine whether it is a schizophrenic or depressive psychosis or a toxic organic one. Our preliminary estimate will determine the gates and pathways open to the patient in these initial moments of contact.

If the picture is predominantly one of confusion, disorientation and loss of memory, organic psychosis should be suspected. If the hallucinations include sensations of crawling bugs on the skin and visual hallucinations are especially evident, a toxic psychosis is possible. We should inquire about drug use. The amphetamine or speed psychosis is almost impossible to distinguish at first glance from the acute schizophrenic psychosis. When there is a suspicion of organic or toxic psychosis, we need to route the patient through a medical or psychiatric service, for this may be an emergency.

The acute depressive or schizophrenic psychosis is always a crisis. If our preliminary assessment leads us to conclude that such an acute psychosis is evident, we should take immediate action. Have the client brought in immediately or convene a crisis team and get to the patient. With enough support, the acute psychosis need not be alarming, but if we suspect the presence of suicidal or homicidal features, we may well have a psychiatric emergency on our hands. Such conditions may require a hospital or well-staffed clinic. If we must see the acute psychotic patient in our private office, we ought to insist on the presence of a responsible relative. We also should have a co-therapist or other colleague present.

1:9. Taking the Next Step

We now have some information. Perhaps it is evident that we are dealing with an emergency. If so, we must get help—*now*.

If it is a crisis, we may try to handle it by telephone. But we may also have to intervene and go to the scene of the crisis. Not all crisis calls require a home visit, though, and the persuasive mental health worker will urge the people to come into the office.

One of the first problems that we encounter in bringing the client into the clinic lies not with the client, but with the staff and the facility. There may already be a heavy case load. One more client today is just too much. There is no one available for an appointment. The psychiatrist must see patients on the first visit and he is here only on Mondays and Thursdays. We look in the appointment book and shudder. Must this client wait a week, two weeks, a month? This, too, is a crisis of sorts.

The case load can rapidly become unbearable in private practice or a small clinic. But if we make ourselves available for crises calls, then we must also make arrangements for immediate and reliable service, whether this involves assigning people to crisis duty or setting up a system of reciprocal referrals. In the outpatient or mental health clinic, someone should be assigned the duty of screening and initial intake, and this person could then be available for crisis cases.

2. First Assessments

There is only a relative difference between the rapid initial telephone appraisal and the first face-to-face interview. The one most obvious difference, however, is that we gain more information by being able to see people and spend more time with them. Clients can see us as well and relate to a person as opposed to a voice on the telephone. The first interview provides us with the opportunity to establish rapport and a working relationship.

Chapter Topics

2:1. Which Clients Do We See Alone?

In routine initial assessments the mental health worker will often face the client alone. But there are situations, such as emergencies, crises, or states of potential violence, when a co-therapist or consultant should be present. There is also the question of interviewing the client singly, the spouses jointly, the immediate family, or a larger group of involved people for the initial interview.

Frequently, we have little choice in constructing the first session. We may be making an initial face-to-face contact following a crisis telephone interview. A group of very upset people may arrive with the designated client-to-be. We see right away that we can't handle the situation alone. Or often a parent or spouse brings the client in. These relatives expect to be included in the interview as they typically have opinions to offer and wish to see what the interview process involves. To ignore them would be to lose a valuable opportunity to learn more about the problem. It is also possible that family members may refuse to participate so that the client appears alone for the first interview.

Despite these conditions, we will have some control over the setting in some situations. A little urging or taking of control when an appointment is being made by telephone can encourage family members to appear with the client or can encourage the client to arrive for the appointment alone.

When we do have a choice, we can select from three kinds of settings for the initial assessment:

1. interviewing the client alone;
2. interviewing the client and the relatives separately;
3. interviewing the assembled group as a unit.

The setting we arrange will reflect our therapeutic orientation and bias the results of the assessment in a particular direction.

There are probably two situations in which the mental health worker sees the client alone even if relatives are present. In the first of these the client asks or otherwise indicates a wish to speak without other family members present and the interviewer has reason to believe that the relatives are dominating, controlling or scapegoating the client. A private interview is, therefore, definitely warranted. Later, it may be important to bring the family members together for these very same reasons, but in the first session it may be wise to concede to the client's wishes. In the second situation the client-to-be is a young person who has moved out of the household or is planning to do so. There is no indication of psychosis and the therapist is inclined toward long-term insight therapy. Many therapists find it advisable to see this client alone and may even refuse to talk to the relatives.

Some mental health workers prefer to see the family as a whole no matter what the situation is. In fact, they would insist on convening the family for the first interview, not just to make an assessment in common, but to establish the actual therapy group for future sessions.

Whether we see an individual client or a family group or a group of affiliated clients becomes, then, a matter of *circumstance and orientation*. In the traditional therapies it was considered desirable to relate to one client. In the new family approaches, the family is the client. With this difference goes a difference in the nature of explanation of the locus and the nature of the problem. In the traditional view, the problem is in and of the individual, the client. In the family view, the problem lies in the family relationships, and it is unwise to accept the label that one family member *is* the problem.

2:2. The Initial Interchange

The client or the family has arrived. They are waiting for us and we must prepare for this first interchange, as it will shape what comes later.

Whenever we engage in any kind of communication, we make a presentation of the self. Consciously or unconsciously, we make statements about who we are and what we are with our bodies, faces, clothing, our total person, as well as our voice. In working with people we must always ask ourselves: Do we present a picture of the harassed, bored, or unconcerned bureaucratic type? Do we look official, slightly worried? Do we scowl and project our jaw as we approach the client? What is our manner of entrance? Do we swagger into the waiting room, approaching the client with a touch of arrogance? What style of clothing do we wear and what is our hair like? What is the manner of our smile? Are we only an official representative of the health establishment or are we there to assist people who are asking for help?

By the same token, we will also notice the clients as we approach. Is the client manacled between two policemen? Is one member of the group inattentive, slumped over and motionless? Or does the client hasten forward to meet us and start the complaints even before we have introduced ourselves? First appearances can be deceptive. A broad smile may reflect good manners or it can be the starting point of deceit. Perhaps the client's smile states simply his gladness at seeing a helping person. We will appraise and reappraise many times in the course of the interview and succeeding therapy.

It is time to say something to the client. Do we say, "Hello, my name is Dr. Jones?" "Mrs. Jones?" Or, shall we say, "I am Mary Jones. I'm the psychologist here"? What about simply identifying oneself as "Mary"? The degree of formality or informality varies with each of us and we must find that mood that fits our comfort as well as the client's. The address, "Hello, Paul. I'm Dr. Jones," is a form traditionally fitting the medical model. It does not, however, add to the helping relationships. Any introduction should be bilateral. "And you're Mrs. Smith?" Or, "Mr. Galento, I'm glad you could come also."

What do we say after we have said hello? Woody Allen worried about this question; how we ease into the problem will not be an insignificant act. "Now, what is the problem?" sounds very officious. "Why don't we move into the office and, maybe, Mr. Galento, you could tell me what happened yesterday?" With experience, the opening remarks can be geared to fit our initial impression of the clients and their problem.

2:3. Framing the Interview

Much of our training directs us to pay attention to certain verbal and nonverbal cues. But there are other elements as well that frame the interview and help define the character of the proceedings.

Chairs, the decor, the degree of privacy and the place itself are important features of the frame. They may denote a calm, hectic, or even emergency atmosphere. They offer a cue to a formal or an informal relationship. The office arrangement may place the interviewer in a clear authoritative role, as is exemplified by the interviewer taking a seat in a large executive office chair and directing the client to a smaller, straight-backed chair. A circle of chairs of equal size or two chairs facing each other suggests a setting of relative egalitarianism. The dress and manner of the interviewer make such statements as well. The white coat, business suit, or casual wear tells a great deal about the form of the proceedings.

How a family sits is important too. The therapist is likely to sit on a chair at one end of a semicircle or at one end of a rectangular arrangement. At the other end a co-therapist may take a chair or, if there is no co-therapist, the most dominant member of the family is likely to sit there. Then those embers of the group who are most closely allied are likely to sit next to each other. If we permit the family to sit as they choose, we have some immediate cues about the family organization.

Sometimes a client or a parent will begin to tell the family's story before everyone has settled in. But, more commonly, the participants take seats, assemble their belongings, take up particular postures, and look to the interviewer to begin. In traditional psychoanalytic interviews, the therapist often avoids taking this role, placing the first statements back on to the patient. More recently, it is common for the interviewer to initiate a round of introductions and briefly reiterate the purpose of the conclave.

If one watches closely, instead of just listening to what is said, an interesting occurrence can be observed at the beginning of the interview. All of the participants will move about in their chairs. They will change postures, light cigarettes, swing their legs or feet, and so forth. Further, they will do so together and keep doing so until they achieve a synchrony of movement like musicians about to begin a concert. When similar positions and synchrony have been achieved, there is usually a moment of silence and immobility, as if the musicians are awaiting the fall of the conductor's baton. The participants have now come into the same space and the same time frame. This brief moment usually passes unnoticed, but it is a signal, no matter how fleeting, that they are ready.

The clients look to the therapist and the therapist looks back, gives an audible cue, such as a clearing of the throat or an "aah," and addresses the first statement or question: "I would like to find out more about the problem," or "What sort of difficulty are you having?" *Consider to whom this opening comment is made, for it defines the therapist's notion of family roles.* Some interviewers recognize this and refuse to address an opening question to any particular member of the group. Yet they unconsciously may focus their gaze on or orient their body toward a particular member. They may move their hand toward one person in the group, while seemingly addressing everyone present.

Distance is an important feature of the relationship as well. In

British, British-American, and Black-American cultures, a face-to-face distance of less than three feet suggests intimacy or high involvement in the relationship. So does touching. In other cultures, such as Hispanic, Italian-American, and Eastern European Jewish traditions, the conventional distance separating discussants is less and they may sit closer, even under rather formal conditions. There may be a great deal of touching as well. What is intimacy to one people, then, is standard informality to others. To label a New England Yankee as cold, distant, standoffish, or defensive is as ethnocentric as calling a Puerto Rican flirtatious, an Italian-American excitable, or someone of Eastern European Jewish descent pushy.

Distance may not be just a matter of culture. Professionals who have been involved in the therapeutic process will use distance as part of their tactics, either consciously or unconsciously. Some therapists sit as far as possible from the client and lean backwards in the chair with an immobile face and crossed arms. Others lean towards the client, hunched forward in a manner of high attention. Some even touch quite troubled clients or sit next to them in a side-by-side position, a common means in our culture of establishing alliances or offering support. Some interviewers are stone-faced; others nod and smile encouragingly. These differences in approach reflect, to be sure, the personality of the interviewer. But they can also reflect therapeutic style. *Learning to vary distance, posture, and bodily orientation provides the therapist with more leverage in practicing better mental health.*

2:4. The Form of the Relationships

It will work to our advantage to appreciate those behaviors that help form a relationship.

Facing the speaker is a common feature of our culture. In a family or group interview the therapist may find himself turning first to one member and then another as each offers an account of the problem. Occasionally, a particular family member holds forth, insisting on being the spokesman for the others. A therapist may have to intervene, interrupt, even point this out as part of the problem. But sometimes the therapist is an unwitting partner in this asymmetry. Without realizing what he is doing, he may address most of his questions to this person or keep looking at him, thus reaffirming his floor rights and his position within the setting.

The angle at which the chairs face each other is important, especially in one-to-one interviews. A 90-degree right angle placement is a relatively informal setting in our culture. A full face-to-face chair placement commonly is an arrangement characteristic of courtship and confrontation. We may select a right angle or full face-to-face settings for strategic purposes, but we should be aware of what we are accomplishing in so doing. Ordinarily, an intermediate angle of 45 degrees provides the kind of flexibility fitting our cultural standards.

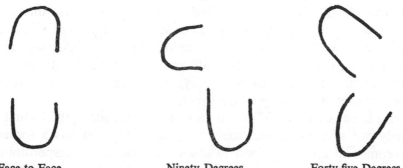

Face-to-Face   Ninety Degrees   Forty-five Degrees

It may pay, for example, to be reserved with a sexually seductive or paranoid client. But it may be important to move towards a frightened, tearful, or depressed person.

Situations alter cases, and our approach initiates and cues the other person to what we are trying to accomplish. If we expect the client to carry the burden of exploration and understanding, we sit back and listen. If we plan to intervene in an active or supportive program, we move in and get started. In a family interview, for instance, we may sit side-by-side with the person we think needs the most support. We may speak a great deal to the others, but our position and bodily orientation state clearly what we are doing at that moment. Obviously, such an overt act on our part will help direct the course of the conversation and determine the kind of interpretations we will be making.

2:5. Guiding the Interview

During the assessment, information must be obtained and the interviewer must have a format for obtaining it. We think that this is the case even in the first session of insight therapy. The first interview should cover the complaints, the history, and the present situation, and conclude with a plan for further action. During the interview, time must be budgeted, topics shifted judiciously, and participants prodded to move with the format. Consequently, we believe that the interviewer should always be in charge of the event.

This is not easy. The client has a format too, even if the format is simply one of evasion and cover-up. The family too has a format. Sometimes all are determined to absolve themselves of responsibility and guilt. Sometimes they try to focus all the blame on one member with the notion of focusing the treatment on, or obtaining hospitalization for, that member. Sometimes they air old arguments and try to get the interviewer to take sides. In these situations, we suggest that the interviewer allow the client or clients to take the lead for the first 20 minutes. While they hold forth with their say, the interviewer gains an excellent opportunity to watch the family in action. Then, after this time period, the interviewer should move in. He should sit forward, interrupt, and quietly and persistently insist on exploring the history and the setting.

Sometimes the movement of the agenda or establishing control of the situation is not the main problem. Rather, it is the quality of the relationship which troubles us. The client or a family member will not talk at all, or he may speak in monosyllables or in a surly, evasive, or openly angry manner. Or perhaps the person keeps questioning the procedure, saying that the process is stupid, wasteful, and useless. Occasionally, a client will insist on using the time for irrelevant purposes like seduction, intimidation, or trivial gossip. *At these moments, we become quite aware of the fact that we have two tasks.* We are to collect information *and* we are to establish a workable relationship. We may find that we will have to postpone or revise our information agenda and take time to deal directly with the relationship and with the quality of the rapport.

We need not always openly state our concern that the relationship has taken a bad turn at this early stage. We can first check the seating configuration, especially the distance between ourselves and the client, the formation of the seating arrangement, etc. We can check our own voice tones and other voice qualities and try changing them. We can check on the attention we are giving to the subject. We can move forward or back. A quiet smile, a casual remark, even a joke may work to defuse the situation. Personal stories that relate to the content often help break the ice and make the interviewer seem more like a fellow human than a bureaucrat. We may find that we will have to change track several times and take several positions before finding one that works to advantage.

Sometimes it is wise to overlook minor disturbances in feelings about the quality of the relationship and stick to the agenda. The trouble can be resolved and the relationship improved in later sessions. But if there is no way to get to a closing plan for the future or if there is reason to believe that the client or family will not return for another try, a crisis has thus developed in the interview. In this case the relational problem must be met head on and explicitly. The interviewer can say what he thinks this problem is and ask the most negative or disruptive person to deal with it. In some cases, though, we will have to accept the fact that there is nothing we can do.

2:6. Eliciting the Complaints

In the jargon of medicine, we say that the client has symptoms. In everyday language, something bothers the client. There is a disturbance of mood, a depression, an unexplainable elation, a great anger or panic. Sometimes there are somatic complaints, such as headache, blurred vision, palpitations, sexual dysfunctions, or gastrointestinal discomforts. And sometimes things do not go well. The marriage is a failure. It is not possible to find a job. Some clients come in with complaints that are self-diagnoses: I am a masochist. I have an oedipus complex. I fear a psychotic breakdown. But some clients do not complain, except perhaps to tell us what others have said about them.

In a family interview the members are likely to complain about each other, about a particular faction, or about one member. We will end up with an inventory of complaints and countercomplaints and we can visualize the dysfunctions and troubles from various perspectives.

Since some clients do not offer complaints or symptoms, we must ask about them. If we are to gain a comprehensive view, we do best when we have an ordered means of proceeding.

We begin by encouraging the client to tells us what most bothers him and then we round out the picture. We can ask about moods, then about bodily functions. One way to gain a broad picture is to start at the top of the head and ask about headaches, vision, hearing, eating, and so forth. We can then turn to the problems of the rest of the body. The next step involves asking about thinking, habits, daily life and relationships.

We want to learn what the client ignores, as well as what he features. But we are not simply dealing with what a person complains about. We want to know more about the sort of person we are talking with, and we want to gain a picture of the assets as well as the difficulties. So we inquire into these matters as well.

As we seek a broader picture of the client, we must watch him carefully. We are not solely creatures of words and we cannot expect a client to verbally articulate all parts of a problem. We must learn to assess mood and its reflections. We learn to observe immobility or hyperactivity. We can witness autonomic responsivity in pupils, skin color, perspiration. We hear speech qualities as well as words—words can be bitten, spat out, and clipped off. They can be murmured in flat monotones without any evidence of caring about them. Clenched teeth or a sigh may accompany statements and tells us something about what is being said. Frowns, giggles, or tears convey meaning at least of equal importance with the words being spoken.

2:7. Obtaining the History

In teasing out the time element, we should work backwards. Are the complaints recent? Do they indicate a change, possibly even a change for the worse? Have the difficulties long been part of the client's life? Are they persistent or episodic? Do they occur only in particular contexts?

We must be especially circumspect with clients who are not familiar with psychodynamic thinking, for a quick jump to early childhood experience may cause a great deal of resistance. So we probe backwards, step-by-step: How long have these things bothered you? Did you have these troubles before you married? How about when you were a younger man? Did you experience the same problems as a teenager? What about when you were a child?

When we have gained a picture of the development of the difficulties, we can then widen the perspective and pursue the broader spiral of personal development in relation to others. We can go into the marriage, parents, work, school. With each set of relations we can also pursue the time factor. Again, we prefer starting with the most recent relations and working backwards, carefully fitting the various pieces of the puzzle together as we go along. As we listen, we relate the symptoms to the history, both personal and relational.

Then we broaden our perspective once again. This time we take a history of the family, beginning with parents, moving to siblings and other immediate and relevant family members and friends. We will want to know where the parents come from, when they came, and what they've done in life. What do they do outside the home? What is their work, activities, and friends? How did the parents get married and how do they get along? What about finances?

In short, we are recommending three increasingly larger circles of knowledge:

1. the problems or complaints;
2. the client and his adjustment;
3. the network of family and friends.

Within each circle we try to gain a sequential narrative of the history. *Histories are important for dealing with the present, and we will want to know what in the past will help us predict the future.*

2:8. Initial Distinctions

We have begun to form some early impressions. We need not make a definitive diagnosis at this stage, but we should start with some distinctions that will determine how we wind up the first interview.

We recommend five broad categories that help us form a perspective of where we are:

I. *Medical Problems*: Is there a suggestion of organic brain disorder, toxic reaction, or a problem with psychiatric medication? If so, we will need a medical or psychiatric consultation.

II. *Psychiatric Emergencies*: Is this client psychotic? This question may not make a difference in a well-staffed clinic or to the experienced therapist as far as referral is concerned. What is critical is whether the psychosis is endangering or not. Is the client suicidal, homicidal, or so disorganized that she may get herself into serious difficulty? If so, hospitalization or immediate medication may be necessary, for we have a psychiatric emergency on our hands.

III. *Crises*: Does it look as though the client is in crisis? Might the client run away, could a terrible fight occur tonight, or could the present problem escalate rapidly and lead to a breakdown? If so, we must once again ask ourselves if we can handle this case, at this moment, alone. Even if we think we can, we may want to ask if we can muster all the client's resources, as well as our own, to carry the person until the next appointment. We strongly urge that a consultation or co-therapist be sought in crisis situations.

IV. *Difficult Cases*: Dramatic and special action may not be necessary, but what if we have reason to believe that this is an especially tough case? Agitated depression is a good example—so are borderline schizophrenics and clients with a history of impulsive behavior or addiction. We will do better in these cases with a supervisor or co-therapist.

V. *Normal Cases*: There are no "normal cases," but there are those that we are certain we can tackle by ourselves. We have made a preliminary diagnosis, formed a tentative plan, and now we make an appointment for the next session.

3. Assessing the Larger Situation

We are gaining an idea of the kind of client we will be working with. But as we proceed in this first interview, we will have to continually reassess our opinions.

If a person habitually presents a schizophrenic picture, we can say, yes, he *is* schizophrenic. Or if our client has a long history of addiction and overdrinking, we can be sure we are dealing with a case of alcoholism. But many cases are not that clear.

The problem may not be just *in* the client. A family may be all too ready to brand one of its members a culprit and thereby absolve other family members of any part in the problem. Yet, *there are instances in which schizophrenia, drinking or depression is in the family system.*

We strongly argue for assessment of *both* the situation *and* the nature of the client's relationships, as well as of the personality problems of the client. We may find ourselves working with, or at least temporarily faced with, a whole network of clients who contribute to the definition of the problem.

Chapter Topics

3:1.   What Has Been Done in the Past?
3:2.   What Is the Life Situation?
3:3.   Provocative Relational Problems
3:4.   Background, Class, and Money
3:5.   Am I Ready, Willing, and Able?
3:6.   How Do I Feel About This?

3:1. What Has Been Done in the Past?

As we gather a history of the client's problem, the client or family members may tell us what has been done about the problem in the past. In fact, he may tell us only a long story of previous treatment and psychotherapy to the point that it is difficult to find out what sorts of maturational experiences he has had. But however we obtain it, it is wise to find out about the history of what has been done.

The fact that a client has had a great deal of psychotherapy before should not discourage us from continuing it. Maybe we can do better, or possibly our work with this client will add to what has been done before by taking the person a step further. However, it could cost us dearly if we dismiss past efforts lightly and consider our predecessors incompetent or uncaring.

There are more immediate reasons to gain a picture of what has been done before. We wish to know what seems to work and what does not; further, we need to know what the client or the family considers worthwhile. Persistent failure of past efforts may be accompanied by feelings of hopelessness about the present and the future. Such feelings may be very serious in a depressive person.

We must also assess what we have done and what was covered in the course of the interview as we look for cues about what might work. Is there anything that we have said which brightens the client, elicits a smile, or provokes a show of hope or interest? We should observe whether or not the client has become less isolated, less unhappy or less uncomfortable as the interview has progressed. If so, we can assume that a hopeful relationship may be unfolding. If not, we may have before us a highly isolated, depressed, or very negative person who will not allow any help to break through the barriers. However, we must keep in mind that it may be our conduct of the interview that is evoking the client's pessimism. It may be time for us to review our approach.

3:2. What Is the Life Situation?

During the course of the interview we must learn who lives with the client. The exact composition of the household and the relationships of the members will prove important, especially as we attempt to understand the problem and begin mustering the supports.

We will also want to inquire about larger circles of relatives and friends who can be called upon for support. Who can usefully be brought into the household to help out and stay with a depressed, lonely or mildly psychotic person? What about parents, siblings, grandparents, uncles or aunts? And what about friends? We need to find out how these potential allies feel about the client and how responsible they have been in the past.

Is there someone who would take in a furious spouse, thus giving the situation a chance to cool down? And, if so, will suspicions and jealousies be given additional fuel in that setting, thereby putting greater strains on an already strained marriage? Perhaps someone suggests that the client take the vacation. But we should be aware of the dangers of the advice. Maybe someone should accompany the client. Loneliness or an unsuccessful attempt to form a relationship with a stranger has precipitated more than one suicide. Moreover, an early schizophrenic psychosis can be escalated by social isolation and separation.

There are other features of the life situation which should be examined. Is the client employed? Where does the client live? Is the household near public transportation? How does the client get to work or to the clinic? Is the neighborhood dangerous? Will a person who acts strange upset the neighbors? Will a mildly psychotic person be attacked? Will the client be afraid to return home after an evening appointment?

3:3. Provocative Relational Problems

If we are psychodynamically oriented, we will assume that the client has had serious relational problems in his developmental years. Otherwise, we will reason, he would not be in this plight today. While taking the history, we have probably gained a glimpse at what we think the problems are. We intend to explore them in depth as we begin an insight or relational psychotherapy program. But this matter of past relational problems is not our primary concern at this point.

What we want to know now is: *Are there ongoing relational problems which are severe enough to precipitate a catastrophe before the next session?*

The following three examples illustrate the importance of gaining a picture in the first session of the severity of any relational problems.

1. Betty has threatened to leave her husband, Joe, who in turn has threatened to beat her if she does. We want to know if Betty will carry out her threat and leave before we have had a chance to discuss the crisis more thoroughly in the next therapy session with the couple. We also want to know how real Joe's threat is.

2. Susan says she hates her mother. They spend hours together arguing. We learn that if her mother doesn't find some excuse for criticizing her daughter, Susan will do something to precipitate an argument. This seems to have been a long-standing pattern between them. We also learn that occasionally an argument ends in Susan's having a psychotic episode. We try to find out what is psychotogenic in those arguments. When we ask about what is said and done, we learn that, after one of these particular arguments, one of them walks out of the house. We then work on the idea of the twosome holding together, with no walkouts, until the therapeutic plan has had a chance to get underway.

3. Charles gets on pretty well as long as he takes his medicine and doesn't drink heavily. We, of course, want to keep Charles sober and on his medication until we have gotten him into a therapy program. We

want to know if he will do it and if his wife, Louise, will help. So we ask Charles *and* his wife about their habits. In the process we discover that Louise sometimes hides his medication, giving it to him only in return for help around the house. Charles, on the other hand, retaliates by drinking. This is going to be a problem for us to deal with and we know from experience that it will take time. Right now we will try to work out a deal with Louise and Charles to maintain the medication routine until the next session.

3:4. Background, Class, and Money

The first session is drawing to a close. There is much more we would like to know, but we must make judicious use of the time remaining.

A great deal of the education of psychotherapists involves training in the psychodynamics of intrapsychic processes. However, as we look more at the character of relationships, a strong familiarity with cultural and class rules will be necessary.

It is valuable to obtain a brief cultural and social history during the first session. Many of us have had some introduction to the differences in family organization. We may recognize the contrasts in the regular and usual ways of doing things as ethnic and social lines are crossed. Jewish-American, Black-American, Irish-American, and Puerto Rican families differ greatly in how they approach, define, and solve problems and how they deal with deviance. Relatives will act toward psychotic family members pretty much as they have been raised to act—and that difference persists in spite of public education and television. Different cultures have different attitudes towards medicine as well.

Social class, too, will make a difference in values, attitudes and a readiness to accept psychotherapy. Changes of class membership often precipitate a crisis or form part of the picture in a personal or family crisis. A sudden promotion or improvement in job and a move to a more affluent neighborhood may seem desirable, yet such changes can foster a separation reaction or a profound sense of guilt and disloyalty. By the same token, the threat of a son or daughter to abandon a middle-class life-style by dropping out of school or moving in with a lover of poor background may instigate a horrible family battle and a consequent psychotic break.

These matters will have to be explored in more detail in other sessions. In this first session, we want an idea of the immediate relevance and importance of these considerations.

There is one more issue to cover before the session closes. What about money? Who has the finances and will they be willing to spend the sums necessary for treatment? We think Mary needs hospitalization, for instance, but neither she nor her parents will consider a public hospital. Are there funds for private hospitalization? If the treatment of choice is psychotherapy, who, if anyone, is willing to pay the costs?

We may hesitate to take up the matter of finances at this first session, for our training leads us to focus on psychological or relational problems. If we work alone in private practice, we will have learned to diplomatically let people know what the costs will be. But what if we work in a public facility? There are costs there, too, and the therapist must make these clear to the client.

3:5. Am I Ready, Willing and Able?

We have looked at the larger picture of the client's situation. Now, before we end this session, we must look at ourselves.

First, do we have the resources needed to take this case? A medical and psychiatric evaluation may be necessary before medication can be prescribed and therapy started. Can we see that this is done? Do we have the time to follow through, since we know from experience that clients may not take care of such matters themselves? Perhaps the client should be hospitalized and we don't have authority to arrange it. What should we do?

Second, there is another aspect of our resources. Can we crowd one more case into an already busy schedule? Such a concern may not matter. If we work in a large clinic, everyone may be busy. In private practice we have the option to refer the client elsewhere, but all too often we do not exercise this alternative.

Thirdly, a willingness to accept this case depends on other factors as well. Perhaps this kind of case bores us; perhaps we have learned from previous experience that we have difficulties with this type of client and problem; perhaps older women are just too difficult for us to treat; or perhaps the man's authoritarian ways irritate us and we find him terribly condescending. All of these factors must be considered before taking on a case.

3:6. How Do I Feel About This?

We must step back and ask, *"How do I feel about this situation?"*

One Saturday a group of visiting planners was being taken on a tour of a large urban hospital. When the group reached the psychiatric emergency ward, they began to ask the admitting officer questions about admitting practices. He explained that he sometimes admitted patients and sometimes sent them home. He was asked how he decided when to admit a patient to the hospital. He thought a while and then said, "I admit them when I feel afraid of them."

We should make use of our feelings. In the initial assessment, we may have developed a feeling of rapport. Perhaps this feeling will persist and our suggestions will be taken. Or perhaps an optimistic feeling and the sense of hope have prevailed throughout the session. Maybe this desperate client will hold on now until we see him again. *If such feelings about the session or relationship are absent, we must be very careful in reaching our conclusions.*

We cannot ignore our negative feelings either. If we are leaning towards hospitalization or referral, it may pay to ask ourselves what reasons justify this decision beyond the fact that we do not like this client.

When we still are not reasonably sure, we have another recourse. We might ask a colleague to assess the client too. Perhaps our consultant will have more experience and fewer doubts about what to do. Then again, perhaps the same doubts will persist.

One part of clinical experience is knowing how we feel. If our consultant isn't sure either, that should not totally discourage us. We have not tried to work alone and we have sought advice. We will make the best recommendation we can. Few mistakes are totally irretrievable.

4. Recognizing Medical and Psychiatric Problems

It may become evident to us that the client is physically ill or psychotic. If so, we have to consider a physical examination, the possibility of hospital admission, or the advisability of medication.

The mental health worker who has not been trained in medicine or psychopharmacology is not empowered by law to make decisions on such matters. Nor is the nonmedical person responsible for making a diagnosis. But there is a responsibility to recognize medical or psychiatric problems and to obtain a consultation from the appropriate specialist. The psychiatrist must also not forget to be alert for medical and neurological problems.

Chapter Topics

40

4:1. Is This Client Physically Ill?

As we are taking the history, we listen and watch the client with another dimension in mind. Could this person have a serious and acute physical illness?

A great many physical illnesses are associated with weakness, easy fatigue, weight loss, and a general feeling of poor being. Cancers are an example. Anemia occurs in people who live alone and eat poorly. The anemias may be manifest in shortness of breath, weakness, rapid pulse, and anxiety. Thyroid overactivity produces an anxiety syndrome. In acute infections the individual will be tired and weak. General aches and pains, chills, fever, and often a headache may accompany infectious conditions.

Severe and lasting headaches are a problem. Tension headaches are usually felt in the back of the neck and across the brows. Severe one-sided headaches suggest a migraine. If a severe, lasting headache is made worse by coughing, vomiting or straining at stool, and the headache is associated with drowsiness or impaired consciousness, it is possible that there is pressure on the brain from a tumor, hemorrhage, or brain injury. The client should be questioned about this possibility and an immediate medical examination should be recommended.

An unexplained paralysis of any muscles needs a follow-up. Double vision, a weakness of one side of the face, a weakness in chewing or swallowing, or a loss of sensation in any region of the body demands a neurological consultation. So does vertigo or dizziness.

The psychotic patient may be seriously run down from lack of food and fluids, sleeplessness, or exposure to the elements. We must watch for the same conditions in the alcoholic and the drug user.

4:2. Chronic Medical and Drug Problems

Some clients will be all too eager to tell us about their physical ills. Their condition may not represent an emergency, but we will want a clear idea of their physical health before we begin a program of psychotherapy.

Diabetes is one illness we will want to watch. The client probably is aware of his condition, but attention will have to be given to certain symptoms. Light headedness and sudden loss of consciousness may result from too much insulin. An early coma can also occur with high blood sugar. *These are emergencies.*

Hypertension is another common illness among older psychotherapy clients. Hypertension may also produce some impairments of consciousness, chest pains, shortness of breath and headaches. In such people, stroke and heart failure are possibilities. In addition, hypertensive people are often on medications which may produce difficulties in combination with antipsychotic medications.

Severe psychosomatic disorders, such as asthma, stomach ulcer and ulcerative colitis, may require psychotherapy and medical surveillance at the same time.

The senile patient is likely to show a general slowness of thinking, loss of recent memory, problems of alertness and orientation, and episodes of depression and paranoid thinking. The arteriosclerotic client is more likely to have headaches, attacks of dizziness, moments of disordered thinking, and loss of orientation.

Often people with long-lasting pain have become addicted to pain-killers. They may seek to gain such medications from a mental health clinic. There are other addictions that may cause a person to seek drugs from the mental health worker. Although the barbiturate addict is less common these days, we should be alert for this kind of case. Usually, barbiturate addicts experience severe insomnia, hypochondriacal symptoms, and a mild tendency to stagger. They look pale and dull in appearance. Today, we more commonly find Valium addictions, in which the client complains mainly of anxiety attacks and conceals the wish for Valium.

4:3. Toxic and Drug-induced Psychoses

A toxic psychosis is critical and may be difficult to spot. It can resemble a functional psychosis like schizophrenia, but it is a medical and neurological emergency.

D.T.'s (Delirium Tremens) is an example. It can occur when one has been drinking heavily for days or weeks, but it can also develop when a drinker *stops* drinking. It often looks as follows: The individual will be very irritable and agitated, will experience sleeplessness, will not be able to sit still, and can be very aggressive. Most spectacular in this picture are visual hallucinations, often of a particular kind. Snakes, rats, or bugs are seen. Especially common are tactile hallucinations or sensations of bugs or ants or the like crawling on the skin.

In acute alcoholism the hallucinations are likely to be auditory. But we must be careful in dealing with hallucinations. Schizophrenic people also experience hallucinations and their appearance can be almost impossible to distinguish from amphetamine psychosis. LSD, angel dust, cocaine, and other drugs also produce a psychotic picture. Substances containing methyl alcohol and sometimes heavy metals that have gotten into the bloodstream can produce a toxic psychosis.

If we suspect a toxic psychosis, we must get some quick answers from the client: Has he been drinking? When did he stop? Is he on drugs?

We don't always get satisfactory answers when we ask the client. Sometimes a relative or friend can help. We can sometimes gain information by calling an agency where the client has been treated in the past. We might notice needle marks or find concealed drugs or liquor. We must use every clue, but first of all we must be alert to the possibility.

There is another kind of problem that requires our attention. A sudden loss of consciousness can be due to a serious brain disorder. Perhaps the client was lethargic, drowsy, occasionally irritable and sarcastic, and experienced difficulty staying with the questions. It is possible that the loss of consciousness is due to exhaustion resulting from days of sleeplessness during an acute pyschosis. But this is not usual and we must be alert—the client may have taken an overdose of barbiturates or he may have sustained a head injury.

Convulsions, partial paralysis, and loss of consciousness are dramatic and they prompt us into action and remind us to ask the client or relatives about drugs or alcohol use. But we should also incorporate these questions into our general history-taking, for the more dramatic symptoms may not occur during the interview period.

4:4. Acute Schizophrenic Psychoses

The acute schizophrenic psychosis is a more common problem for the young mental health worker than toxic or drug-induced psychoses. Such cases are usually referred to a clinic or hospital, but they appear in private practice as well. So important is this syndrome to the mental health worker that it will pay us to recognize the pleomorphic manifestations—the many different forms—of this condition.

Some Examples

Cathy seems sane enough. It is her husband who brings her to see us, complaining that she just sits and stares. Cathy denies any voices or visions and has no complaints herself. We notice that she is very quiet and does not want to talk to us. Her answers are vague, evasive, and monosyllabic.

Lee has always been a quiet, hardworking young man. This morning he suddenly slapped his baby, threatened his wife, and ran screaming from the apartment. When he came back he was in panic and his speech was incoherent. He does not seem to know where he is or what day it is. He looks quite bewildered.

Sharon is restrained by both her parents and her brother, for she is trying to run out of the consultation room. She has been up all night pacing the floor and screaming out the window, cursing the neighbors. She says we are devils who are trying to kill her.

James has been brought to us by his father. He refuses to talk and sits facing away from us. Finally, he accuses us of plotting against him. Then he falls silent, but he makes facial grimaces of a strange nature.

Mary is singing. She refuses to sit down. She paces about the room bragging about her exploits and threatening her mother at the same time. She laughs in a silly, giddy manner. She says she feels fine and has no problems.

Sue has no obviously abnormal behavior and no complaints. She tells us that she has been psychotic in the past and is now experiencing the confusion she knows so well. She asks us for some medication.

4:5. Perceptual and Thought Disorders in Schizophrenia

Some schizophrenic clients have obvious disorders of thought and perception. They claim they are being persecuted, followed, punished, or plotted against. Things look different to them. Familiar faces seem somehow distorted. Noises in the room are given special and strange meanings. Conversations on the street are about them and the radio announcer may be talking about them, too.

Some acute schizophrenic clients have auditory hallucinations. They hear voices which may order them to harm themselves or to take aggressive action against other people. Often the voices insult, berate or blame them. Less common these days are visions of sacred or frightening things.

Sometimes there are hallucinations of body changes, smells, or skin sensations. Be careful here. If the tactile hallucinations are especially prominent, the condition may be a toxic psychosis. Also, if the hallucinations of smell and taste are more prominent than auditory hallucinations, the possibility of a temporal lobe tumor should be considered.

But not all schizophrenic people have these disorders of perception. In fact, many clinicians regard delusions and hallucinations as "secondary symptoms" of schizophrenia. Yet, even when these disturbances of external perception are absent, one finds a problem in the "internal sense" of space and time. The client may be unsure of times and dates. He finds it difficult to remember what happened a minute ago and what happened earlier. His words may tumble out in improper order. Thoughts ramble on and do not follow the usual order of narration. There are tangents, interruptions, and alternative lines of thought. The total flow of events and the sense of spatial organization get mixed up. Boundaries are unclear and fuzzy, including the boundaries between the self and others. Distance seems askew and the client will find it difficult to say what is up close.

In short, the sense of perspective is lost and there is a disturbance in the client's sense of space and time.

4:6. Emotional Fluctuations in Schizophrenia

The schizophrenic disorder in perception and sequential thinking is associated with a loss of emotional modulation. Moods and feelings seem out of control. There is extreme anxiety or uncontrolled rage. The intensity of emotions may be out of keeping with the situations which provoke them. Or the emotionality is said to be inappropriate altogether—we see no *evident* cause for the emotionality.

There are other feelings in schizophrenia. Elation and depression may occur. Also, the mood may change rapidly. Sometimes the emotion of the moment seems contrary to what we would expect. An angering remark is greeted with laughter. Strong affects are not under usual cognitive control.

Yet, the very opposite picture is characteristic in schizophrenia, too. The client may show *no evident emotion at all*. There is only a dull, apathetic disregard for what is said and what goes on. And on occasions, situations which we would expect to result in an extreme emotional outburst do not seem to touch the client. There is no joy at a happy event and no remorse or crying at a profound loss.

We judge these emotions in part by the tone of the voice and by facial expressions. But there is also a general disorder of the muscle tonus of the entire body in schizophrenia. This disorder, like other emotional manifestations, is either too much or too little—some schizo-phrenic people sit motionless, limp and flacid, like wet dishrags, while others are in constant movement. The face is a mass of tic-like move-ments, the arms and legs are continuously repositioned, the body is tight, the eyes are darting, and the client needs to run or pace.

In our culture there is yet another basis for the judgment of emo-tionality. When people carry out tasks such as explaining themselves in a cool and logical order, we think of them as cerebral or rational. When their ability to sequence ideas and emotions is disordered, as in schizophrenia, we think of this as a failure of emotional control.

In general, schizophrenia is characterized by some lack of emotional modulation.

4:7. Relationships in Schizophrenia

In the acute psychosis the client may be extremely withdrawn. He may refuse to talk to anyone and even flee or run away. On the other hand, some clients cling. They hold on to a relative as if in panic. Or they follow the clinical staff, begging for explanations, pills or attention of some kind. As in the case of emotions, relationships in schizo-phrenia present a puzzling paradox of opposites.

The history of social adjustment shows some of the same extremes. The client was always a loner, remaining significantly apart from others, and rarely engaging in social interaction. Conversely, the client might have been overly outgoing, almost desperately so, before the psychotic break. Some schizophrenic people are overly compliant, while others are overly rebellious.

The family history often indicates that the client has always been exceptionally dependent upon a single person, often the mother, while he has been distant from the other family members. This is the symbiotic picture of schizophrenia. But when the schizophrenic person reaches the teen years, the close partners often become alienated. Each will avoid the other or express a great deal of mutual disagreement, hate, or blame. Then the symbiotic relationship becomes ambivalent. In some cases there is no history of overdependency, and the withdrawn, secluded characteristics we witness today have prevailed since childhood.

There is usually a lack of social skill in most schizophrenic clients. It is not only that they avoid relationships; it is also that they have little ability to form and hold them. They are either too remote with other people or they crowd them, both figuratively and physically. They say too little or they become garrulous, bristling, or badgering. Either they stare at you or they avoid meeting your gaze altogether. The facial expressions are strange and misleading. There is very little gesturing. Often the schizophrenic person has no greeting behavior and no courtship behavior of a normal sort.

In short, the relationships of the schizophrenic person are abnormal and so is the ability to form relationships.

4:8. Endangering Schizophrenic Pictures

The acute schizophrenic psychosis is always an emergency. Support, medication, or hospitalization may be necessary. But the recognition of an acute psychosis is not our only consideration. *The first problem is whether the psychosis is endangering.* Will this client commit suicide, attack someone, or get into a dangerous situation?

In part these possibilities are learned from the history. If there is a history of previous psychotic episodes in which suicidal attempts, homicidal threats, fleeing in panic, or getting into dangerous situations have occurred, then we can expect that these may occur again. Or if the present attack has included any of these features, we must plan for the worst.

Often we obtain no such history from clients. They conceal such matters from us or they are too confused to tell us about them. In this case, we can try to contact others who might be able to provide the needed information—a relative, friend, roommate. Thus, *we probe for a history of violence or endangering behaviors.* We may have to ask, for instance, what instructions the voices give in order to assess how dangerous the instructions might be if carried out.

We do not rely on what we hear alone. We make observations for ourselves. We try to gauge the facial and bodily behaviors as evidence of hostility, resentment, and suspiciousness. We test judgment and impairment of orientation. A markedly confused client can get into danger quite inadvertently. We inquire about dangerous thoughts, threatening hallucinations, and violent feelings. *And we watch what the client does* as he talks about such matters or declines to discuss them.

4:9. Depressive, Suicidal Syndromes

The depressive client usually tells us about the mood of depression: "I am sad, hopeless, unhappy, or depressed." And the client looks it. His face is drooped in a mask of sadness and immobility. His body is hunched over, sagging, immobile, and slow of movement. There is a loss of appetite and usually marked insomnia. Body functions are disturbed and underactive. Typically, the client blames himself for everything.

It is not enough to recognize the depression. We have another more pressing question to answer. *Is this client potentially suicidal? If there is any hint of this possibility, this is an emergency.*

The question is not easy to answer. A profound pessimism and a sense of hopelessness and helplessness often cue us to the danger of suicide. So should a marked and unexpressed rage. A failure to show any hope or interest in the interview or in a promising treatment plan is not a good sign.

It is also important to determine whether there is a past history of suicidal preoccupations and whether there is a history of suicide in the family. Sometimes depressed clients copy someone else who has recently committed suicide. We have also found that suicide is a traditional means of solving problems in some families. This is true in certain cultures as well—Scandinavia, Hungary, and Japan are examples. *We must not guess about historical precedents. We must ask and find out.*

There is another problem in the depressive states. The depression may be masked by marked overactivity and agitated restlessness. Or the depression may not appear, but instead there is a manic picture. The client is grandiose, pseudo-elated, though anxious, belligerent, jocular in gallows humor, but quite hyperirritable if he is frustrated.

To make matters more complicated, the acutely depressed or manic client may have delusions, hallucinations, and other evidences of psychosis which resemble schizophrenia. In fact, the differential diagnosis is difficult or impossible at times.

But when there is danger of violence or suicide we need not waste our time with a diagnosis. We take emergency action.

4:10. Start the Ball Rolling

If it becomes evident in the initial interview that there is a medical or psychiatric emergency, there is no point going on with a protracted exploratory interview. A consultation is needed and we may as well start the ball rolling. Before we take this step, *we want to shift from the tactics of interviewing and replace them with measures that increase the client's trust in us.*

We begin first by establishing a greater measure of rapport with the client and family, for we will want their cooperation with our planned action. We say things like: "We realize what a strain this has all been." We empathize with the severity of the problem. We offer brief reassurances, even while we unfold the idea that the problem is serious enough to warrant a consultation.

How we manage the move from interviewing to actually getting the consultant will depend on our feelings for the situation. We can excuse ourselves, saying we wish to consult with a particular person and then step out of the interviewing room. Or, as soon as the client or family begins to accept the idea of a consultation, we pick up the telephone and place the call.

Follow-through. If the client must go to another location for the consultation, call, arrange for it, and follow up to make certain it occurred. The very sick or endangering psychotic client cannot be left to wander about the streets or hospital corridors unattended. If there are no family members or friends to get an irresponsible client to the right place, either take him yourself or find someone responsible who can.

5. Making Plans and Getting Started

Experienced psychotherapists tackle almost any problem on an outpatient basis, though they may carry the case in cooperation with colleagues and family members. The newcomer to mental health must be more careful. Advice and support will be necessary for the difficult cases, and we must learn to make use of them.

Chapter Topics

53

5:1. Emergencies Need Psychotherapy Too

The fact that we must call in medical or psychiatric help does not mean that psychotherapy is not necessary. There are at least three situations in which we do psychotherapy before and while emergency measures are being taken.

1. *We may need to do psychotherapy to gain the cooperation of the client or family.* The client may be terrified of hospitalization and we will have to reassure, explain and possibly persuade. *But* we should not use lies and tricks to force an admission. In another case, the client has to be cared for until a medical consultation can be arranged. The illness may be so acute that we have to stop the assessment procedure and try to form a relationship in order to relieve the anxiety while we wait for help.

2. Perhaps the client is hospitalized as part of an emergency routine. The mental health worker is a member of the hospital staff and will conduct psychotherapy during the period of hospitalization, because *psychotherapy is important in acute psychosis.* In fact, it is often possible to circumvent hospitalization altogether if adequate psychotherapy can be provided.

3. There are instances in which medical or psychiatric consultation is necessary. In some of these cases we may keep primary responsibility for the client and continue the psychotherapy program during the course of the consultation and during the period of medical treatment.

5:2. Medical Supports for Outpatient Therapy

A psychiatric backup may be useful in treating clients with severe anxiety or marked insomnia problems. In such instances, it may be necessary to give the client some symptom relief until changes in the emotional state and the life situation can be brought about with a regime of psychotherapy and education. A psychiatrist may prescribe valium, some other minor tranquilizer, or a sleeping medication. It is important to avoid long-term use of these habituating drugs and to have a physician watch for adverse effects.

The chronic medically ill client, such as an individual with asthma, diabetes, or hypertension, may need both medical regulation and psychotherapy. The epileptic client will require our particular attention. In epilepsy a medical routine involving an anti-epileptic drug, such as dilantin, may be necessary, but the issue of epileptic manifestations can be complicated and unclear. There are epileptic syndromes of a psychomotor type in which grand mal convulsions do not occur. Instead, the client has episodes of sudden and seemingly unprovoked rages, or overreactions to minor frustrations, coupled with very impulsive antisocial behavior. When one has a client like this in psychotherapy, it is wise to ask a physician to see the client and consider the use of an anti-epileptic drug.

5:3. Family Supports for the Disturbed Outpatient

Many psychotic clients can be carried in psychotherapy as outpatients after a period of hospitalization or in the place of hospitalization. We should muster what family supports there are or help the client find a social network other than the family. In these instances, the social supports bolster the individual psychotherapy and medication regimes.

A first step in mustering social support networks is to interview the client about which relatives or friends might be helpful. Then a meeting is called of those who are willing to attend. At this meeting the problems of the client are discussed with the client present. Confidences can still be preserved while attention focuses on what the others can stop doing and what they can start doing that might be more helpful.

We can picture levels of increasing support:

1. At the level of minimum support, key relatives or friends agree to allow the client to visit them on occasions and they promise to help the client with certain economic, legal and everyday matters. For instance, a cousin may agree to help the client find a better apartment and then help him move. An aunt might be enlisted to make certain the client is never completely out of food and money and that the house cleaning is not totally neglected.

2. At a level of greater support, family members and friends may agree to provide the client with a place to live in their homes, or find a suitable alternative and contribute towards the living expenses. At this level, the relatives also agree to have occasional meetings where they are coached on how to optimize their support and improve their relationship with the client.

3. At a maximum level of support, the family members agree, for a time at least, to take on total round-the-clock responsibility for the client. They are to offer reassurance, protection and comfort and, if necessary, they are to help prevent suicide. The mental health worker has the responsibility to train, coach and support them in this effort.

5:4. Supports for the Crises of Passage

Every human being passes through certain life crises, such as birth, puberty and death. Each culture also identifies other moments and marks them as significant cultural events. Marriage is an example. Here in America these passages often become crises. Examples are starting school, reaching adolescence, leaving home, becoming divorced and facing death.

As mental health workers we soon learn the long list of such crises of passage. In a figurative sense we can lump this list under two kinds of problems.

1. There are those crises that clearly and immediately involve two or more people and all parties know it. Marital conflicts, divorces, and battles involving children and parents are examples.

2. Then there are those crises that seem to involve just the single individual. Either this person lives alone without close friends or relatives, or the relatives disavow any responsibility for the individual's problem. When faced with this latter case, the therapist *and* the client must decide whether to go it alone or whether to put pressure on

relatives in order to get them more involved in the client's behalf or to at least include them actively in a family or network therapy program.

It is not our intention to form a dichotomy between crisis situations and personality disorders or mental illnesses. Some clients always have severe problems with adjustments *and* feelings, while others have manifest problems only with a change of status. Others only experience problems when they face a bad situation. But the differences here are relative. *Psychotherapy between crises will help a client meet the next one. Help and support during a crisis can result in learning how to meet and deal with difficult situations.*

In practice we will find that we must meet a crisis before we can conduct a long-term therapeutic program, because the client does not come to us until the crisis has developed. Consequently, we begin the process of therapy and we try to muster what supports there are to deal with the present crisis. We have supervisors, consultants, co-therapists, and, hopefully, the relatives and friends of the client to help us through the moment of crisis.

5:5. Relational and Family Crises

There are many reasons for trying to bring in close relatives or friends for an attempt at family and relational psychotherapies. However, two reasons stand out and are worth attention:

1. A client simply is not able to make an adequate life for himself.
2. The client and the parties concerned should continue to live together.

Examples of the first instance would be the chronically psychotic, the deficient, the disabled and the medically ill. Examples of the second type would be a child or a spouse when the couple intends to remain married.

It is often the case that spouses, friends and other family members are unwilling to participate in a therapy program. *But when there is resistance, the problem might well be the orientation of the psychotherapist.* Some therapists prefer individual therapy, or they do not know how to do family therapy, or they consider it unimportant. If the therapist's heart is not in the effort to convene a network of family members or friends for joint therapy, the attempts to do so will probably fail.

In the case of a marriage that has the potential for continuing, certain characteristic crises may initiate marital therapy. These crises may in and of themselves be superficial, but they may also present evidences of more deeply rooted problems. *In any case, the crises are the manifest difficulties and they should be dealt with in their own right.* Frigidity or impotence, infidelity, chronic arguments, violence, battles over careers, and battles for control and domination are examples of such crises.

Family crises are prone to occur at various stages of development of the oldest or the youngest child. For instance, fathers often withdraw as their daughter reaches the age of four or five and again when she reaches adolescence. Often mothers and sons grow closer together while fathers grow progressively distant from the spouse and the son.

There are other points of family crises, for example, when children grow up, leave home, get seriously ill while away from home or get married. There are family crises at retirement, at the death of one parent, at the birth of grandchildren. Also, there are family crises that have no apparent relation to the age and passages of the children or parents.

5:6. Enlisting a Co-therapist

It is customary to call in a co-therapist in dealing with certain kinds of family problems. A prime example is the family with a schizophrenic member. In such families a single therapist can get lost in the heavy, dull and negative emotionality of the family. There are bizarre mythologies. Talking the case over with a co-therapist can help overcome the family's obstacles. Moreover, co-therapists can share responsibilities for the client, check upon each other's objectivity, and cover for each other when one must be absent from a session.

Group therapy often involves a co-therapist. Having two therapists present is almost mandatory in doing group therapy with upset and unreliable psychotic patients on the ward. It is necessary for the large meetings of therapeutic communities in the hospital ward as well.

These are the usual settings for co-therapy. But why not do co-therapy with any client or in any situation if there is sufficient staff? Two inexperienced co-therapists can learn from each other and offer more to the client at the same time. Before and after each session they can meet to discuss different or similar impressions. They can monitor each other's involvement. The presence of a second therapist can help prevent one's being consumed by the client, a common problem with young and inexperienced therapists.

It is also a valuable experience to *watch* someone else do psychotherapy, even if that other person is inexperienced. One cannot see one's own face during the session, and one rarely pays attention to one's own body. The dimensions and impact of nonverbal behavior become conscious to us when we watch someone else doing the therapy. Needless to say, much can be learned in co-therapy by watching an experienced therapist. Being there at the same time is much different from discussing the academics of the case after the hour.

5:7. Supervision for the Tough Cases

Certain syndromes are notoriously difficult in one-to-one psychotherapy. It may be wise to spot these cases and arrange for supervision or help from the beginning. Seeking such assistance from the moment of the first interview will avoid discouragement later and may prove to be a valuable learning experience as well. We will discuss three examples of such difficult cases.

1. *Schizophrenic types are difficult.* Psychotherapy for the acutely psychotic outpatient is a harrowing, exhausting and tense business. Get help. The chronically psychotic client may have flare-ups of a disturbing nature. The paranoid client may endlessly argue with us, criticize and thwart our efforts, and distrust whatever we do. But the main difficulty may be the degree to which we and the client become discouraged with the lack of progress.

The chronic schizophrenic can also be very compliant and over-dependent. We will be expected to do everything for the client. Our strongest efforts to wean him and encourage him to become active and mobile may be of little avail.

Borderline schizophrenics can also be difficult. They may be passive and resistant to change. They may learn to trust and work with us, but they accomplish little outside the sessions. It takes skill and some aggressiveness to move these people.

2. *The depressive client is usually frustrating.* The risk of suicide is an early worry. The clients may know how to hold this risk over our heads as a means of control, making us feel guilty and responsible for their actions.

The lifelong depressive is slow to change. Just as the therapy experience seems most promising, he gets worse. This paradox maintains the dependence on therapy. It will take some risky confrontations to break these impasses. Under such circumstances it pays to have experienced coaching.

3. *The impulsive and antisocial cases are hard to keep working.* These clients fail to show up just at the moment when we think that progress can be made. They may telephone us at any time, make an unreasonable request for us to bail them out of trouble, and then blame us if we do not comply. Addicts and alcoholics often present this kind of difficult behavior. In addition, they can add to the problem by showing up for an appointment intoxicated or they can spend their time with us attempting to obtain drugs.

5:8. Evoking the Supports of the System

Co-therapy and supervision may not be enough help for some of the tougher cases. Both the client's network and the supports of the larger mental health system may have to be called upon.

The psychotic client who sees us on an outpatient basis is a case in point. It will be useful if we can find a relative who can be counted on to keep the client out of trouble at night and on weekends and holidays. Often there is just a spouse or parent who is available, for no one else will care. But how do we proceed if this partner is part of the problem, as is so often the case?

Another problem is what to do with the very psychotic client during the day. Most community mental health clinics provide useful alternatives: day hospital programs, lounges, or occupational therapy programs. The client can come in, join the program, and take time out for a private therapy session. Sometimes the client can be enrolled in school or a special rehabilitation or educational program. This will provide daytime supervision and also promote the goals of maturation and learning. This still leaves the problem of supervision at night and on the weekend.

The client who lives alone can present some difficulty for us. Loneliness and depression mount at night or over a long holiday weekend. This may lead to a critical incident involving the police, crisis intervention, or physical injury. Consequently, if family cannot be mustered to help on a regular basis, special living arrangements will have to be made. Foster home care, a nursing facility, or boarding house arranged by a day hospital may do the job.

Some clients are so difficult that the staff of an entire clinic gets involved in their support. They show up for psychotherapy when we have an appointment with another client. They upset the day hospital, scare secretaries or other nonmental health staff and start fights with other clients. Eventually, all of the staff gets to know them and, when their therapist is busy, whoever is free will spend time with them. From a psychoanalytic perspective, we might worry that such interference would dilute the transference, but with very disturbed clients, we will be glad for any help.

5:9. Referring Special Cases

There are some problems that require referral, not because these cases are too hard or too dangerous to handle alone, but simply because there are other people and other places that are likely to provide a better service for the clients. These clients have particular problems that require a special kind of care that most mental health workers are not trained to provide.

The alcoholic and the heroin addict are cases in point. Sometimes it is simply impossible to do outpatient psychotherapy with someone who is drinking or drugged. Referral to an alternative facility, such as a hospital setting where detoxification can be safely carried out or where special medications can be regularly monitored, will be the practical solution. There also are programs, including Alcoholics Anonymous and various drug centers, that offer community and group work which is more appropriate to the individual's problem.

Speech defects are another problem requiring special referral. Aphasics, stammerers, stutterers and other individuals with severe speech problems should be handled by experts in this field.

5:10. Handling This One Alone

It seems that we have reviewed an endless number of instances in which we need psychiatric, medical, family or colleague support. Are there no cases we can tackle alone? After all, it is enjoyable for just the client and therapist to sit together, and there is a time when we should take full responsibility for a case on our own.

The great majority of people who come to a clinic or a private office can be seen in psychotherapy without medical or other supports. Further, a great many crises and psychotic episodes that regularly end in hospitalization could be handled in outpatient settings with a bit of advice, experience, and a proper setting. The acute psychosis, for instance, responds well to psychotherapy. A new and meaningful relationship can be formed and the client has a chance to break from home or reliance on institutions. To many people, a psychotic break can be a blessing in disguise, for it brings them to help for the first time.

The usual and ideal client for one-to-one psychotherapy will have a neurotic problem. As we bring the assessment interview to a close, we see no reason not to take the client on an outpatient basis. No special supports seem necessary. It is thus time to get started.

II. Working with the Problem

There are many treatment approaches in mental health and it is not easy to know which would be the best to use with a particular client. We suggest one *choose that approach which may help the client most, rather than that which will be acceptable to some doctrinal school of thought.*

There is a rough rule about the selection of a psychotherapy: The more disorganized the client, the more directive the therapy should be. At one end of the spectrum we find rigid, hyperorganized people. For them we may choose an expressive, insight approach. At the other end are disorganized adolescents and psychotic people who are severely lacking in the ability to organize thoughts and modulate emotions. For them we need methods which enable them to achieve direction, order, and more stable relationships. Some clients, however, are both rigid and unstable. And some clients change as time passes or when they experience a crisis. We, too, may have to change our approaches.

As we work with more disturbed clients who are in turbulent crises, we not only modify our methods of pyschotherapy, but also add additional approaches and means of supports. In psychosis, for example, we may add medications, activity programs, family therapy, and group therapy to our program of treatment. In the clinic or the hospital, a client may be in four or five treatment procedures at the same time. The therapist becomes a case manager as well as a psychotherapist.

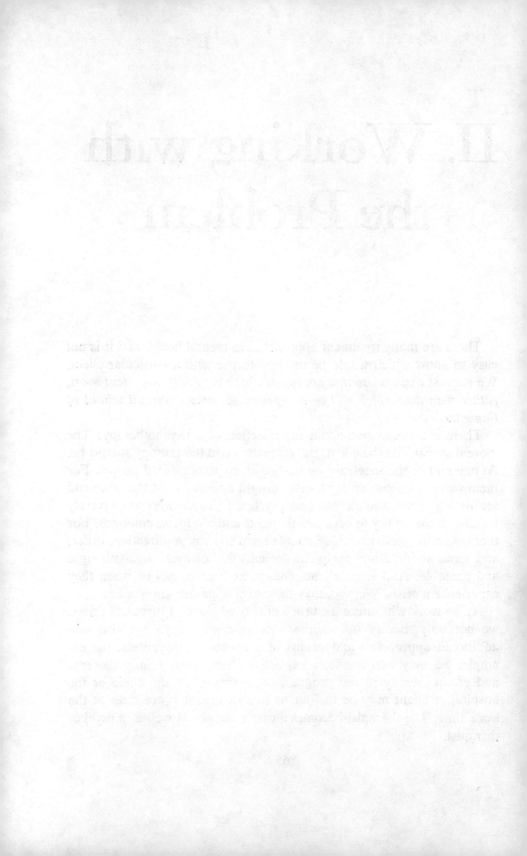

6. Participating in the Therapeutic Alliance

The relationships formed in psychotherapy will depend in part on the kinds of people who form them. Since both the client and the therapist function in the relationship, who they are will influence the character of that relationship.

But the shape of a relationship is also dependent on the goals and methods of treatment. In insight therapy, for instance, the therapist should keep her personality at a low profile and allow the client to transfer past notions to the therapist. But in active or directive therapy, the traits of the therapist may be accented and used as techniques in the therapy itself.

Chapter Topics

6:1. Being and Being Present

Being

The therapist is not a technique. The therapist is a woman or a man who is young, middle-aged, or old. The therapist is huge and commanding or tiny and unpretentious. The therapist is of British, Jewish, Italian, African, or Hispanic descent. And so on. These are the realities. They are not concocted and they are not concealable.

In a psychological sense, a therapist can be authoritarian or egalitarian, aggressive or passive, articulate or unskilled with words. In any session a therapist can be anxious, calm, interested, bored, or preoccupied with other matters. These are elements of being, too. They may or may not be related directly to a particular client or to what that client is doing or saying. *The more aware we are of our psychological being, the more able we are to modify it.*

We can use our states of being as a technique in psychotherapy. We can use what we are to illustrate an idea or we can minimize the impact of our particular characteristics to develop the self-attention in the client. There may be times when it is valuable to discuss one's own background or personality traits. There are other times when we are bored and it may be valuable to admit it. For example, Mr. Jones had been a client in insight-oriented therapy for many months. Among other things he was an insufferable bore. He spoke in a low monotone, repeated himself endlessly, and talked on and on about the same subject. Ms. Smith, his therapist, occasionally dozed off while listening to him and then had to take time apologizing. Should she not have admitted her boredom and worked it out with the client? She finally did and her confession made a difference. At first he was hurt, but as he thought about it, he decided she might have a point and he decided to work on being less boring.

Being There

Full attention and thoughtfulness are owed the client. One listens and watches, uses some techniques when they are called for, and keeps in mind the overall strategy of the therapy. *The therapist should be there for the client.* Mr. Thaler finds himself distracted during sessions. Some clients are boring, to be sure, but not all. The problem is Mr. Thaler, for he is not there. He seems continuously concerned and preoccupied with his marital problems. That is all he talks about when he has lunch with his colleagues. Could that be his problem in therapy sessions, too?

If we persistently and repeatedly have traits and viewpoints which are inimical to our clients and ourselves, it is high time for us to become a client and work on straightening ourselves out.

6:2. The Adoption of Particular Therapeutic Styles

There are several stereotypical pictures of the good or successful therapist. To some degree, all psychotherapists have learned one or more of these professional roles in a more or less conscious way. A therapeutic style can be deliberately copied, practiced, and used. *Often forgotten, however, is the very critical fact that any style, position, or tactic has its uses and its limitations.*

1. *The authoritarian style* is erect, commanding, forceful, and incisive. This stance is fortified with a business suit or white coat, deep voice qualities, and visible tokens of one's certificates, degrees, and honors.

2. *The parental presentations* stress kindness, thoughtfulness, patience, and toned-down authoritarianism. The devoted mother and the kind and supportive father represent positive stereotypes in our culture. They appear as styles in psychotherapy as well.

3. *The wise and learned counselor* relies on uncombed hair, ill-fitting clothing (for both sexes), much looking up at the ceiling, beard or chin stroking, and overattentive listening. It is the academic, the philosopher, style.

4. *The radical peer look* requires slouched postures, blue jeans, and casual shirts and blouses. Long hair and sneakers or sandals are recommended.

5. *The psychoanalytic neutral* calls for nondescript clothing and a remarkable degree of facelessness and noncommittal silence.

These styles are useful for certain kinds of rapport and confidence. But they can be put on in only a limited measure. It is absurd for the middle-aged, experienced therapist to pretend to be a peer or play hip with a teenaged client. It is absurd, too, to carry out directive therapy in a vague psychoanalytic manner. In the long run, any assumed style will become the least of the important qualities we offer to our clients.

6:3. Beyond the Blank Screen

The psychoanalytically-trained therapist has mastered the art of not speaking often. He has also learned to hold a blank face and reduce information at the nonverbal level. But even experienced therapists may not be conscious of other modalities of communication. The following three examples illustrate the importance of this point.

1. *Gaze.* The disciplined psychotherapist does not say anything when the client describes an unacceptable action and the insight therapist attempts to withhold commands and judgments. But what happens when the therapist momentarily stares into the client's eyes? In our culture such a gaze is as commanding as an authoritarian in-

struction. If a therapist consistently looks down or away when a client talks about certain matters, avoidance is clearly suggested.

2. *Vocal qualities and small gestures.* Smiles, nodding of the head, and "uh-huhs" convey information. *They are not neutral.* An unwitting smile suggests approval. An uh-huh instructs the client to go on speaking or suggests an understanding of or an agreement with what is being said.

3. *Timing.* If a therapist smiles and says "uh-huh" when the client talks about certain subjects, but looks away and does not make any sound during other points in the flow of speech, the client will soon be conditioned to focus on certain topics. This is but one reason that "free associations" are not free.

The therapist does not realize how he steers and conditions a client with small behaviors. We can learn more about how we use our eyes and faces by looking in the mirror or asking our friends. However, we don't wish to eradicate the last vestiges of being humanly responsive in therapy. An awareness of our behaviors simply helps us become a better helper.

6:4. Making Sense and Being Clear

Perhaps we are unable to follow the commandments of a particular approach that say how the good therapist should act. Perhaps we cannot sit back, be quiet, and neutral to do psychoanalysis. Then we might do better at some other therapy. Perhaps we are slow and quiet of speech and we find it hard to be directive. We cannot be all things. But there is one maxim we must obey in any approach: *We have to make sense.*

For one thing, our actions and our statements should roughly go together. Our dress and posture should approximate our points of view. If we express a belief in certain principles of psychotherapy, these are the ones we should use with our clients. We should try to do what we say and say what we do. If we tell a client we like them, we should do so with a face that looks like liking. What value can the statement have if it is spoken in a bored monotone with the face and eyes averted? If we keep reminding a client that certain scatological expressions are inappropriate, we must stop grinning as we make the disapproving statements.

We must learn to speak in a comprehensible manner. It does not help to look at the ceiling and mumble out an interpretation. If we cannot speak distinctly, clearly, and comprehensibly, then we should practice doing so. If comments roll off our lips in monotone, mumble, or whispered hesitancy, we are not being effective.

Finally, when we say something important to a client, we should watch and listen to be certain that we have been understood. If there is doubt, we should go over it again—and then again if necessary.

6:5. Sharing Feelings and Viewpoints

The neutrality of the insight therapist officially continues throughout the course of therapy. This noncommittal stance may develop into a total way-of-life. The young insight therapist may come to make love, discipline the children, and hold a conversation with friends as if he were conducting an insight hour. One may need to relearn how to smile, argue, and react emotionally again.

A prominent psychoanalyst tells the story of a young woman patient who came in one day in tears and said, "I cannot stay for my hour. My father just died and I have to catch a plane right away to get home." The analyst violated a traditional rule of non-involvement. He put his arm around her, a human and comforting act, and walked her to the office door, saying, "Call me when you get back." *There are times, even in insight therapy, when it is important to break technique and share a human interaction. One of these is a time of crisis. Another is the end of the course of treatment.*

In more active, directive therapies we often share feelings with the client. We acknowledge that our flushed face, jutted jaw, and clipped words are, indeed, evidences of anger, annoyance, or embarrassment. And we may discuss what has made us angry. Or we might admit we have a cold and feel terrible. If we attribute our negative feelings to the client's behavior, we can say why. If there is another source for our mood, it will be a relief for the client to learn this. *In most learning experiences, life's usual reactions should not be hidden.*

Some therapists share their own experiences and points of view. They can thus provide a philosophy of life and some examples of how to do things. In so doing, they also foster a sense of sharing.

6:6. Analyzing the Relationship

In most psychotherapies the relationship of client and therapist is itself a focus of examination, but there are different ways to achieve this end.

In the insight therapies, the analysis of the relationship is often the major focus. The expectation is that the client is to relive in the therapy relationship experiences he has had in childhood. When the difference between old expectations and the actualities of the therapist-client relationship have been distinguished, we say that the "transference is resolved."

In the psychotherapy of highly reserved, overly independent, and distrustful clients, it may be important to guide the client into a discussion of the therapy relationship, for such people may try to avoid the subject. They may even deny that they have any feelings for the therapist.

It is deleterious to a psychotherapy of any length to ignore the relationship of therapist and client. For one thing, a great many angry feelings and unrealistic ideas can accumulate without being dispelled or clarified. Consequently, the relationship can be endangered. A failure to deal with the relationship is the loss of an opportunity to learn about this critical dimension of human interaction.

For these reasons the therapist may direct the client's attention to such matters: "How do you feel about me?" "You seem annoyed. Does that have to do with me?" "You've been coming here for several weeks now and not once have you mentioned how you feel about me." "Do you think I've been a help?" "Why are you so hesitant to talk about how you feel about me?" "Why don't we talk about the two of us?"

A time-honored psychoanalytic technique can be useful at this point. Instead of first stating our opinions of the client's feelings towards us, we start by pointing out how the client is avoiding the subject. Thus, we talk to the notion of defenses. This gives us a basis for further exploration.

6:7. Insisting on Limits

Many psychotherapists wish to be egalitarian and non-demanding, but there are two issues where we must take a firm stand.

1. *Insisting on discussion and participation.* In the lingo of our trade we are not to "act out." We should not take impulsive and adversive action without considering and discussing that action first. We must try to find out what motivates our decision, how we feel, and what actions we might take as a result of a decision. *We should insist in therapy that the client avoid impulsive or half-baked courses of action as well.* Our clients should be instructed to come in and talk over problems and possible actions before they act.

Some of the current therapies do not feature self-examination. Instead, they focus on relationships or interactions. But the rule still holds. We insist that our clients take a hard look at their relationships and talk them over before taking any potentially damaging or harmful action.

2. *Insisting on limits and non-exploitation.* The therapist is not to exploit the client or the client's dependency or transference in order to take revenge, charge excessive fees, gain sexual titillation, and so on. The therapist must also insist that the client not use the therapist or the therapy in similar ways. The limits of the therapist's tolerance and service are defined by the strategy of the method. They must be explained to the client and maintained during the course of the treatment. If the limits have to be changed to meet an emergency, crisis, or special situation, this act must be explained and made comprehensible.

It is also valuable not to permit a client or a therapeutic relationship to exploit other people, such as a relative or supervisor, or the clinic or agency.

6:8. Crises in the Therapeutic Alliance

Sooner or later a crisis is likely to occur in the therapeutic alliance. Three common examples are described below.

1. *The crisis of whitemail.* There can be two very attractive clients. One is the client who is pretty, handsome, personable, talented, or highly intelligent. The other is the client who shows a rapid improvement. The development of the therapy relationship in such instances can result in whitemail. These clients reward us so much that we are inclined to do extra little things for them, make special appointments, stay overtime, become devoted. The problem comes when we try to stop. Clients may do anything, including threatening suicide, to make us continue this special relationship. It is usually only at this point that we become aware of those extra steps we have taken for them.

2. *The crisis of blackmail.* Blackmail usually begins modestly and can be quite subtle at first. We are late once for an appointment and the client talks of suicide, but we do not recognize the connection. At another time we refuse to see him in the evening and he threatens to stop the therapy. The pace mounts rapidly. If we do not take over more of his life, suicide will be threatened again. The next thing we know, he insists on living with us or else he will die or become psychotic again.

3. *The crisis of separation.* When we agree to terminate the therapy, a crisis often occurs. The client accepts the decision and then shortly thereafter suffers a relapse with a return of the symptoms. There is depression or perhaps a suicidal threat. We give in and continue the therapy.

It is always dangerous to allow oneself to be exploited, at any level. We may go on and on, feeling quite devoted, self-sacrificing, and humanistic. But sooner or later we unwittingly take our revenge, in one form or the other. We forget the appointment or find reason to terminate the treatment. *We can avoid such unpleasant incidents by remaining steady in our commitments.*

The crises of whitemail and blackmail call for more drastic measures. The client may, indeed, have another psychotic break or a dangerous depression when we attempt to strongly define the limits. We need to deal with this directly and decisively, and this means taking risks. If we do not, we run a risk that the relationship, based as it is on blackmail, will go on and on without improvement. If improvement is to occur, we must challenge the client on his use of threats and relapses to control us. *At these moments we need the help of an experienced therapist.*

6:9. Not Being Scared

There are crises in the therapeutic alliance. We learn to deal with them, partly by experiencing them and partly by seeking help and advice.

There will be crises outside the sessions also. Often the young therapist lives in fear of a suicide or a tragedy occurring when she is not there. At times it may even reach the point of believing a disaster will occur *because* she is not there.

We must face the brutal fact that sooner or later we will experience the worst. Someday a client will commit suicide, get hurt, or run away. And someday it will happen because the client couldn't reach us. All we can do is take reasonable safeguards, convene a support network for the difficult client, have someone cover for us when we are away, and ask for help when we feel scared. *We cannot be miracle workers.* The therapist is human and tries to do the human and commonsense thing.

When our client does become psychotic, it may be less tragic than it seems. A psychotic episode can be a blessing for some who merely exist in life. The psychosis becomes the first chance to reach competent help, to heal, learn and grow, and to get a new start in a better setting.

In the past, there was a widespread myth that a patient would become psychotic *because* the therapist made the wrong interpretation. We don't believe it! *In our opinion clients do not become psychotic because of what a therapist said.* People frequently do become psychotic during therapy, but usually the break occurs when a persistently contradictory relationship has developed from which they cannot gain improvement or release. Sometimes people get psychotic and enter a crisis state when confronting separation or some form of exploitation. These situations, however, grow slowly and the therapist has time to spot them and get help.

Sometimes psychotherapy is scary, for some clients are scary. Sometimes it is boring and depressing. But sometimes it is exciting, especially after we have overcome our anxiety about doing therapy.

7. Doing Insight Therapy

The insight psychotherapies derive from psychoanalysis. They are ordinarily used with people who are neurotic in the broad sense of the word, who have long-standing problems about feeling well and getting on in almost any situation. These therapies are based on the premise that one is released from repetitive patterns as one becomes aware of or gains insight into their childhood origins. Insight therapies are usually carried out by forming a one-to-one therapeutic alliance in which the client is encouraged to remember childhood experiences, face unconscious feelings, and understand how current relationships reflect past relational problems.

Chapter Topics

7:1. The Special Meta-relationship of Insight Therapy

Before one can understand the techniques of insight therapy, one must understand the particular relationship that characterizes the therapeutic alliance. In the terms of communication theory, the alliance is described as a "meta-relationship": The therapist speaks "about" what the client has said or has done instead of responding in kind. To appreciate this idea we must understand how people ordinarily participate in a human interaction.

If two people meet on the street and one says "hello," the other usually responds by saying "hello," too. If one person puts out a hand for a handshake, the other usually does so also. If one person flirts at a party, the other person responds in kind or declines. *Any interaction is usually characterized by people acting in similar and comparable ways.*

But this is not how the therapist acts in insight therapy. He does not answer a question or trade stories and experiences. When the client tells a story, the therapist may be silent or may speak *about the story,* that is, about what it means. In so doing, he moves "meta" to the client's action; he broadens his perspective of the action and makes a comment about it by attributing meaning to it.

Later the client is expected to learn how to take a "meta" position to his own actions and statements, that is, he learns to say or think or remember something and then tries to interpret its meaning. But clients who do not understand the purpose of a therapist's meta-response are often confused, hostile, or surprised by it. In everyday life it is downright rude to withhold a response in kind. It can be most frustrating not to receive the advice or encouragement that is being sought.

Many psychotherapists are so accustomed to meta-responses that they forget that many clients do not understand their purpose in fostering self-examination. If the therapist does not appreciate this and interprets the client's negativity or incomprehension as resistance or defensiveness, neither party will understand the other and the therapy will be off to a very bad start. *One must explain a meta-response and its purpose at the beginning of therapy.*

Since the therapist will refrain from responding in kind, the idea must be explained. Then, what is the client's assignment? The client is instructed to say anything that comes into his mind without holding back or censoring. This is what is meant in insight therapy by the rule of free association. This rule must be explained also.

7:2. Patience with Patients

When the therapist has made an assessment, formed a contract for therapy, and explained how insight therapy is conducted, the insight sessions begin. The client is to help in the process, but not take over.

There are several ways that the therapist can assist the client, but *the most important of all is patience.* One has to wait. One has to resist the temptation to jump in with interpretations, encouragements, or criticisms and give the client a chance to talk, think, remember, search, consider, and come up with some ideas of his own.

Patience is critical. If ideas and comments are jammed down the client's throat, they will be resisted. One who is persuaded against one's will remains unpersuaded still. It takes time to cool intense emotions and to listen to what one's self is saying. It takes even more time to think about it.

The therapist may prompt the client: "Can you say more about this?" "Is there anything else you remember?" "Uh-huh, I see. How did this make you feel?" But these promptings should not yet urge the client to an interpretation. They simply encourage the client to keep talking and remembering, with the idea that he should say anything he can about the problem or the event.

7:3. Some Techniques of Insight Therapy

At some point the therapist steps in to clarify or speed up the process of self-understanding. Usually this intervention occurs when the client has had time to review a situation carefully, have it in mind, and recognize that something is unclear or missing. There are common techniques to foster insight:

1. *The Confrontation.* Clients talk around important matters. There are obvious parts of the story they do not seem to grasp. They tell an experience over and over again, but each time they leave out a key dimension. One client tells about a childhood memory, but there is something vague she cannot recall. Who was it? What happened? Another client complains again and again. His boss is critical. His wife sneers at him. His mother was never satisfied. But at no point does he mention anything at all about what he does to merit this abuse. The next client tells about an experience in great detail. But at no point is there even a passing reference to what she may have felt. An aspect is missing.

Sooner or later the therapist must point out what is missing: "I notice that you cannot recall a key point. There must be a reason for that. Did something unpleasant or terrible happen?" In the next case the therapist says, "Let me point something out to you. You always blame other people. Is there something you do in these situations?" Or, "You never mention how you feel. Don't you have feelings about these things?"

The confrontation is made gently. It is often put first as a question, "Do *you* tend to always blame other people?" Later, it may be put more forcefully, "You always blame others, but weren't you furious?" *The art of therapy requires that we time the confrontation.* We wait until we think the client almost sees the point himself, or we wait until evidence makes the point almost obvious.

2. *Making Connections.* We want the client to see the pattern or the entire configuration. We want him to become aware of what happened, who did what, how the people felt about it, and why they have done what they did. Eventually we want the client to see that certain feelings and certain actions are taken by him over and over again. Finally, we want the client to realize that what is going on now is rooted in much earlier experiences.

We try to put it together for our clients and encourage them to learn to do so for themselves as well. We make connections: "It seems to me that being angry is a cause of the dream in which your father was killed." "Could it be that feeling scared was the reason you stayed in bed yesterday and complained of not feeling well?" "You seem to goof up just when you are about to get a better job. I recall you spoke about the same thing occurring at school. Do you remember that?"

3. *The Interpretation.* In the interpretation we not only make a confrontation and perhaps a connection, but we give meaning to it. We give the symptom a frame of reference. This is commonly drawn from psychoanalytic theory, but the theory is not necessarily stated: "Sometimes a man who is very attached to his mother cannot love any other woman." "This breathing difficulty could have begun when you were little, since you were smothered with tight controls all of the time as a child." "Maybe your hidden anger plays a part in raising your blood pressure." "Experiences that hurt in childhood may be forgotten, but they leave a scar and make us fearful of trying certain things later on."

The client may reject the interpretation or politely agree and pass on to some other subject. But when the interpretation is meaningful to the client, it will open up a broader realm of understanding. The client reevaluates old problems and behaviors in the light of the new perspective.

7:4. Interpret the Defenses

In psychoanalytic theory it is believed that we fail to remember because remembering would be dangerous or frightening. Not knowing conceals a forbidden impulse, an unacceptable feeling or a self-depreciating memory. Ways of not knowing are called *defenses*.

All sorts of defense mechanisms have been described. We forget. This is called *repression*. We remember but deny that the event happened or that we were involved in it. This is called *denial*. Or we lean over backwards with contrasting or opposite behaviors in order to hide from ourselves and others that we are inclined in a particular direction. For example, we are extremely kind and considerate so that we unconsciously hide our rage. This is called *reaction formation*. There are many other mechanisms of this kind in psychodynamic theory. *The therapist is to dispel these defenses so that the client can recognize and face what is being concealed.*

There is an Aesop's fable in which the sun and the wind wager to see which can get a man to take his coat off. The harder and more aggressively the wind blows, the tighter the man wraps his coat around him. The sun takes a turn and gently beams down on the man, letting him grow warmer and warmer until he takes off his coat. A time-honored principle about making interpretations in an insight therapy suggests that if one acts like the wind, behaving aggressively and impetuously, the defenses are likely to get stronger. However, if we exercise patience, like the sun, we will achieve our goals. Take it easy. Give the client a chance to face the undisclosed. *When we do point out something, we should interpret the defenses rather than the hidden impulse or unacceptable feelings.* Don't say, "You are a," or "You really want to have sex with your mother." Perhaps late in therapy we will say these things when we are certain the client is already aware of them and needs forceful prodding. But before this point is reached, we must make our interpretations along other lines, on how the client avoids, ignores, stays away from a subject, forgets, and so on. *Interpret the mechanisms by which the concealment is continued and give the client a chance to find out what is being concealed.*

If a client resists an insight or an interpretation, back off—for a while. When the point comes up again, repeat the interpretation, or lead the client back to the point with a question.

The manner of confronting the client is important, too. Don't let an unwitting sneer or condemnation creep in. It does not pay to make a meta-comment with arrogance, as if one were handing down an eternal truth. Remember, an interpretation is an hypothesis that should be stated in the form of a question for the first few times. The therapy session is a cooperative enterprise. It is not a courtroom trial.

As we offer an interpretation, we must also offer reassurance: "It is natural to have such wishes." "Every child feels that way at times." "It seems natural to hate him. He treated you very badly."

7:5. Resolving Transference

The hallmark of a psychoanalytic type of therapy is the living out of transference. In all phases of this form of psychotherapy, the client is likely to transfer to the therapist old attitudes, feelings, and ways of acting. This tendency gradually increases. At times the transferred attitudes become very real to the client and may totally dominate the sessions.

The intensity of the transference may be extreme. The more psychotic types of clients seem to believe that the therapist *is* the mother, father, or sibling of earlier experience. Other clients *feel* as if this is so. Marked dependency, rage, strong sexual feelings, and other very vivid experiences may occur. If the therapist rides through these states without overreacting to them, in time the strong feelings will weaken. The client begins to separate and distinguish these past impressions and stereotypes from the ways in which the therapist actually behaves. In psychoanalytic theory, this "working through" of the transference is considered an essential experience of insight therapy.

Thus, the therapist directs the client's attention to those transferred reactions that are unrealistic. As the therapy continues and the transferred attitudes and distortions increase, these become the focus of our confrontations and interpretations: "Are you treating me like you did your father?" "It seems that you confuse what I say with what your mother says." "Is the anger you just showed towards me the way it felt when your mother did not listen to you?"

But remember, the goal is to relieve the client from transferred reactions that do not fit the real therapeutic alliance. *If the client is to see this difference, it must exist in fact.* We cannot act like the client's father or mother acted and then expect him to resolve the difference. And we cannot expect the client to sort out the realities of the relationship if we act unfairly or unrealistically toward him. We must be aware of our countertransference to the client and avoid treating him unrealistically.

There is a tendency in psychodynamic circles to overwork the concepts of transference and countertransference until they include anything that the client or therapist does or feels. The two parties may like or dislike each other, for instance, for very real reasons. Sometimes the two parties stir up feelings in each other which both blame on transferences. Also, sometimes patterns of action and thought that are characteristic of an entire culture are misperceived as specific patterns transferred from a particular father or mother. For example, a minority group member who grew up suspicious of all majority group authority figures has a distrust of the therapist that is not simply transferred from his relationship with his father.

7:6. Difficulties of Termination

In session after session the client continues to remember, talk, and seek understanding, while the therapist tries to expedite the process with the techniques of the approach. But as the sessions continue, the client should make progress. The client should gain a broader understanding until his life makes some sense. His major difficulties should improve and some progress should be made toward a cherished goal. *If such progress does not occur, one must seek a consultation or a supervisory session.*

The client should become more realistic about the therapist. He begins to disagree with the therapist about realistic points. He begins to make some decisions without help. When this occurs, it is time to consider the prospect of terminating the therapy.

However, when the termination date has been set, a perplexing twist is likely to happen. All of the client's original symptoms return. Is this unexplainable or is it an unconscious attempt to maintain the therapeutic alliance without separation? Since it is often hard to tell, a consultation may prove useful.

7:7. Difficulties of Evaluating Insight Therapy

Improvement is difficult to assess. Any improvement is likely to bring a client into new ways of life and hence into new problems. For example, a client who has been unemployed or who has had only a menial job may become active and proficient enough with the help of therapy to take on a career orientation or win a promotion. This very step brings with it new responsibilities, new challenges and new anxieties, with the consequence of pushing the client back into therapy. Similarly, an isolated and socially detached client who improves in psychotherapy may grow more socially active, perhaps even forming a relationship with someone of the opposite sex. This new way of life can bring new problems to face and deal with.

The problem of assessing improvement and bringing about termination is also aggravated by grand and unrealistic expectations of what insight therapy can accomplish. Both client and therapist may expect a marked and general change in all realms of functioning. The result of the course of therapy has sometimes included the expectation that the client has no more need of the therapist, of any other therapist, or of support and dependency in general. No other important human relationship ends with such expectations. All of us need help, guidance, and perspective in difficult times.

8. Doing the Active Psychotherapies

Insight therapies take months and years to accomplish their goals. Many clients and institutions lack the resources to follow through with the traditional insight program. And some kinds of clients—for example schizophrenic, antisocial, addicted, and very compulsive people —do not do well in approaches that are non-directive. Consequently, shortened, more directive methods have evolved. Often these approaches incorporate some features of insight therapy into other more "active" techniques of support, direction, advice, and persuasion.

Chapter Topics

8:1. Focused Versions of Insight-like Procedures

In some therapies the focus will be on one particular aspect of the problem and expressive techniques, as well as techniques of persuasion, will be used.

1. *Direct Interpretations.* The therapist does not wait for the client to reach the later stages of self-examination in some approaches. Instead, early in the course of treatment, confrontations and interpretations are made in an active and sometimes aggressive way. This technique is sometimes used with clients who have had previous insight therapy and sometimes with clients who are psychotic or in crisis.

2. *Focusing on Aspects of the Problem.* The therapist can zero in on those affects, values, and experiences that seem to be most directly related to the client's main problem or discomfort. For instance, the client may most obviously suffer from headaches, asthma, or a tendency to rebel against authority. The therapist then holds the client's attention on the central problem by repeatedly asking questions about it and by directing the client's associations to those themes that relate to the problem. When interpretations or confrontations are made, they take up issues that have apparent relevance to the focal problem.

3. *Expressive Therapies.* One of the more popular of the active insight approaches concentrates on certain emotional states and on how these are expressed or withheld. In some instances, anxiety and its causes become the focus of the therapy. In others, a failure to mourn a past loss will be the theme of the treatment. Most commonly, anger, rage, and hostility are the subjects of expressive therapy. The goal is to gain an expression of repressed or suppressed feelings. The expressive therapies are employed with various degrees of conceptual sophistication:

(a) In the simplest version it is assumed that the client is sick because he has "bottled up" large stores of emotion. In these "abreactive" versions of expressive therapy, we get the client to express whatever emotion is allegedly held in. The client is encouraged to scream, say angry things, cry, have sex, or whatever. If this encouragement does not suffice, the therapist may employ additional measures, such as teasing, taunting, demanding, or having a group of clients encourage the expression and reward its occurrence.

(b) In more sophisticated versions, the client is encouraged to become aware of various emotions and their consequences on behavior, symptoms, and human relationships.

(c) At a still more sophisticated level, the client should develop an understanding of her emotions and gain social skill in using and in dealing with them.

4. *Adding Persuasion.* Sometimes clients seem to have an adequate insight into their motives and feelings, yet they do not undertake changes in their lives or otherwise put their insights to work. In these situations, some active psychotherapists become more aggressive and add a series of persuasive pressures to the therapy. Clients can be encouraged, pushed, or rewarded for trying to change. Clients also can be teased, shamed, kidded, or taunted into taking a particular step. Some therapists take clients by the hand and virtually force them to try something that they are afraid of, such as riding an elevator or speaking up in their own defense.

Traditional insight therapists discourage the use of direct interpretations, focused areas of concentration, and, especially, active persuasion. In their view, a real and deep insight is achieved with care, and its very achievement frees the client to move forward. Any efforts to persuade, therefore, would impose the therapist's values on the client. Active psychotherapists could argue in return that insight itself is a form of persuasion. When one discovers that he has a distasteful feeling or motive, the discovery itself is a powerful impetus to change. It may be that insight and persuasion are not as different as we might believe.

8:2. Focusing on the Therapeutic Relationship

In a relational approach to psychotherapy, the focus is not on the traits or psychodynamics of the client. Instead, the relationship of the client and therapist becomes a central point of exploration. The client and therapist can discuss the distance or the closeness between them. They can analyze why and how misunderstandings have occurred and talk about differences between them. It is also important for the therapist to remember that people differ not only because they are deviant or pathological, but also because they occasionally differ from the therapist.

In using these therapies, the therapist fosters a relatedness with the client and discusses the client's resistances to forming a relationship. As the relationship develops, its positive and negative feelings are described. Any ways in which the client distorts or misconceives the relationship will also be discussed. Some therapists indicate the similarities in the therapeutic relationship with early life experiences. In short, a relational therapy may feature what is ordinarily the last portion of an insight therapy, that is, the nature of the client's problems in forming a mature relationship.

But in many relational therapies the emphasis is on becoming closely and positively engaged with the therapist. Insight is not an essential technique of the therapy. Everyday, practical problems can be discussed. The therapist may set limits, offer advice and otherwise serve as a good friend, a substitute parent, or a helpful older sibling. In this manner, the therapist becomes a coach, mentor, and model for the client.

At one extreme, a client may simply copy the values, styles, and role of the therapist. At the other extreme, the client uses the therapist as a model of what he does *not* want to be. Between the extremes, a client can learn certain values, mannerisms, and life directions and then evaluate these for himself. Thus he begins to develop his own personality.

A problem can occur in the relationship between therapist and client. The client may feel less distrust, more warmth, and greater understanding and skill *in* the therapeutic alliance, *but these acquisitions may not be carried over into any other relationship in the client's life*. The client improves only during the sessions. A therapist must be on guard for this possibility and encourage the client to use what he has learned in forming and holding other relationships as well.

8:3. Techniques of Support and Direction

Supportive and directive methods are used in the more active forms of therapy.

Encouragement

Some clients need a great deal of encouragement. We explain to them that treatment takes time. We tell them that things do get better and that we expect to help them. It is our job to discover their assets and encourage them positively. We agree with them that they are frustrated and pessimistic and we support them by pointing out that these feelings are natural up to a point. We remind our depressive clients that it is usual during a depression to feel down and bleak about the future. We can praise improvements or positive efforts. All of us need *some* encouragement.

Support

Earlier we mentioned the need in certain situations to muster relatives, friends, and institutions to support the client. *As therapists we, too, should support the client during psychotherapy.* Small acts on our part, such as smiling, head nodding, and commenting, support any new effort or understanding that the client reaches. Sometimes we must also support our client against other people who are unfair, overly critical, or exploitative. Occasionally, we support a client against arbitrary rulings by our own superiors and institutions. We also support a sensible plan to make social contacts, form relationships, earn money, or even fall in love.

Control and Dissuasion

There are moments in active psychotherapy when we must take an authoritarian posture and try everything at our disposal to prevent a client from doing something self-destructive. A teenager may provocatively repeat our statements of support at home and thus risk angry parents halting the therapy. A suicidal client could threaten self-violence. Another discusses with us a plan that could well take him to prison. We have to say something. We warn, cajole, persuade, but we do not ignore. If our efforts do not suffice and we believe the situation is potentially dangerous, then we must call in supports or consider medications or hospitalization. *Our first duty is to keep the client safe and well. Our second is to keep the therapy going.* A colleague of ours used to tell suicidal patients, "If you commit suicide, I'll kill you." Some reacted with a smile in appreciation at the absurdity—and the real concern—of the statement.

Advice and Direction

Many clients in the successful private practice will be quite experienced in life and well organized in their behavior and life planning—too well organized in some cases. But we cannot assume that broad experience and sophistication occur with all clients who come to us. Many clients are naive, unknowledgeable, or psychotically disorganized. We must help them by providing practical knowledge about living and by giving direction for the future. Thus we ask suggestive questions: Have you gone to the eye doctor? Did you ask about welfare? Do you eat meats and vegetables? Have you ever told him how you feel when he does that? Did you try what we talked about yesterday?

We can make long-range suggestions as well and we can then help to hammer out plans for the future. Further, we can help in carrying out these plans by reminding them of the plan in future sessions, making alternative suggestions, and using insight techniques to deal with their inhibitions. We keep certain clients at the task, instead of letting them ramble on in free associations that have been transferred from the figures of early life. In the more active psychotherapies we are likely also to bring our own contributions and traits into the picture. We can encourage our clients to talk about the things we say and do that anger or disturb them. We can work on our differences and our problems *together*.

A time-honored method of forceful suggestion and persuasion is hypnosis. The hypnotist induces the client to accept a dependent, suggestible state of mind that in some cases deepens to resemble a trance or sleep-like state. From this position of authority the hypnotist can suggest that the patient will give up certain negative behaviors, feel better, and otherwise change. Some clients follow such suggestions in an almost compulsive way.

8:4. Techniques of Conditioning and Behavioral Modification

A large number of therapists use techniques which are based upon a model of operant conditioning, i.e., desired responses or behaviors are rewarded while negative, symptomatic ones are discouraged. Many behavioral therapists also employ other techniques such as insight-fostering, suggestion, advice and support as well, but the primary reliance in behavioral modification is upon conditioning.

Models of conditioning derive mainly from the academic tradition in psychology rather than from either the medical model of classical psychiatry or the views of psychoanalysis. This results in two major differences in the concepts and emphasis in behavioral modification. First, behavioral modification emphasizes *educational* viewpoints. Concepts of problem-solving and training are features rather than those of psychopathology and treatment. The emphasis is upon adverse *behaviors* rather than on diagnostic categories, though the concept of "symptom" is often retained in behavioral modification. In some versions of behavioral modification, concepts of human engineering or shaping of behavior are stressed; these terms seem to engage the disapproval of the "humanistic" psychologists, who prefer to view therapy as a procedure in which the client has more choices and a more cooperative role. Unfortunately, negative motion pictures like "Clockwork Orange" have given the impression that conditioning procedures are dictatorial and political manipulations of almost mystical power.

Second, the fact that behavioral modification is not based upon psychoanalytic thinking leads to an emphasis upon the *present* state of behavior and symptoms rather than upon the early life history or etiology of human difficulties. It is argued that historical events cannot be changed but operant methods can be used to alter present difficulties in the current situation. The behavioral therapist might well say he does not care *why* a client hurts or abuses himself. The main thing is to stop it. Once a negative symptom is stopped, a cycle of more positive events can begin and gather strength with further reinforcement.

Technically speaking, it is possible to bring negative reinforcement to bear by aversive techniques or to reward more favorable behaviors or changes in a positive direction. Both approaches have been used in behavioral modification, but the tendency in recent years has been away from the use of punishment and other aversive techniques. B. F. Skinner often pointed out that children had already been conditioned by punishment. He believed that learning was facilitated by rewards rather than by punishment. Most behavioral modification today follows the direction of rewards to strengthen or reinforce improvements or more useful behavior. The therapist and client agree upon what responses would be desirable and then the therapist rewards such behavior when it occurs. In many such approaches the rewards consist of tokens such as coins, poker chips or candies. In some therapies these tokens can be exchanged for more valuable acquisitions, such as hospital privileges. Obviously, the therapist's approval also supplements the tokens as operant conditioners and eventually the respect and approval of other people maintain the behavior.

It is not easy to compare the results of behavioral modification with other approaches such as insight therapy, since behavioral modification procedures are directed at specific symptoms or problems rather than at a personality reorganization. However, it does appear that behavior modification does have positive results with the very types of problems which respond least favorably to insight therapies. Obsessions and compulsions are examples and in phobias behavior modification may well be the treatment of choice.

8:5. Direct Service and Client Advocacy

In one form or another, advocacy and direct service have long been part of helping psychotic and poor people. But these methods have become more clearly defined in the community mental health movement.

The simplest versions of direct service and client advocacy include advice and a follow-up to see that the client has done what must be done. The client is referred, for example, to a helping agency, to a physician, or to an attorney. In more active versions, the therapist goes with the client and directly aids the process of service. The therapist may get a letter of recommendation for the client or help the client fill out necessary application forms. Direct aid is also provided in helping the client find an apartment or get on the welfare rolls. With elderly, infirm, isolated, and chronically psychotic clients, this is often the only means by which these critical life steps are completed.

The mental health worker may also become an advocate for the client. The client might be walked through a complex and refractory bureaucracy. The client might be supported against discriminatory practices and hostile relatives and neighbors. Legislation and class action suits can be drafted and taken to the legislature, courts, or voters. Cognizance is taken of the fact that clients, especially chronic psychotic clients, are a disenfranchised minority in our society.

8:6. Techniques in Schizophrenia

Psychotherapists in private practice used to treat only neurotic patients who were considered good candidates for long-term insight therapies. The troublesome, impulsive, and psychotic patients were sent to a hospital. Private practitioners now see more psychotic clients as outpatients. In fact, since the younger mental health worker will deal with acutely psychotic clients in all sorts of settings, it is important to have some practical guides for the psychotherapy of psychosis.

Gaining Rapport

Often psychotic clients evade and avoid relating to the worker. The first task is to gain a measure of rapport and cooperation. To do so, *one must be there*, regularly and reliably. Sometimes it takes great patience and persistence to establish rapport. We must be able to endure coldness, seeming indifference, and occasional verbal abuse. Psychotics who are paranoid will endlessly test our good intentions and honesty.

There is no use sitting there day after day in silence waiting for the schizophrenic client to like us. *Wade in.* Offer reassurances, affirmations of our goals, and practical help. Try an active dialogue, rebut suspicions, challenge the client to try another relationship. Tell a story about some other unnamed client who was helped; tell a story about one's own fears and craziness. Sometimes a joke can break the ice.

Say something—anything—that might initiate a dialogue. Any kind of conversation helps the psychotic organize cognition and reduce the wild excursions into fantasy and emotion. The psychotic often cannot maintain enough conceptual organization to tell a story, develop a plan, or form a point of view in a logical sequence. *Conversation can help the client to do this.* The content may not be important. *What is important is the active interchange.* The psychotic may become increasingly disorganized and upset if left alone to free associate while we remain silent. Even a mild argument may help if we avoid bitterness and recrimination.

Insight techniques may be useful, too, but we should *be careful. Don't let the client wander off into more and more disorganized thinking.* Interrupt and reinitiate a dialogue to help the client's sense of organization. Do not strip the client of defenses against aggression, sex, or close relationships *until and unless* there is a reasonable chance that he can handle these matters. Moreover, if the client gets into a relationship that is beyond his capacity to handle, a painful failure may be the result. Thus, prepare the client for what we are and will be and modulate the efforts with the situation.

Providing Services

There are little things one can do for the psychotic client. Provide her with a coke or coffee. Intercede with her mother or spouse. Talk to the physician about the pain in the client's back. At this point we shouldn't worry about the psychodynamics of pain or dependency. We are trying to form a relationship with a solitary human who does not know how to relate.

There will come a time for advice, discussion of future plans, and education in the business of living, loving, and working. This time will come when *two things* happen: the client becomes less psychotic and the client accepts a relationship of interaction and discussion with the therapist. *These two changes are not separate. The psychosis will abate when and if the client forms an affiliation with someone.*

Dealing With Dependency

Some psychotic clients do become extremely dependent. The moment they began to think that the worker is reliable and helpful, they will become helplessly and totally dependent on the worker. They will take all of her time, call her over and over again, and do little in their own behalf—*unless and until the mental health worker begins to set clear limits and sticks by them.*

There is a serious problem with forming a dependent relationship with psychotic clients. When and if such a relationship is completed, it is then difficult to terminate it without a recurrence of psychosis. We should be prepared to break with the schizophrenic after inducing him to care about us. The more inexperienced we are, the more we will need supervision to help in the weaning process.

8:7. Doing What It Takes

If we have a private practice with enough referrals, we can afford to be selective, taking certain kinds of clients and referring the others. Perhaps we can hold to one doctrine of psychotherapy and use only that method with all our clients. *But on the front line of mental health, there is no place for doctrinal loyalties or inflexible choices of methods.*

Doctrinal positions about what is "good" psychotherapy or about the "proper" method of therapy are matters for affluent practitioners and academics. Few therapists have the status to say, "I will do only long-term insight therapy." Most of us will have all sorts of clients to deal with. They need support, advice, and attention to their immediate problems, as well as to their broader symptoms.

On the front line, we do what has to be done. There are many approaches and we tailor them to the client and the problem. We put methods together to form an effective overall strategy, for we want to do *what works*. If the chosen technique doesn't work, then we try something else. This may involve shifting from a one-to-one approach and trying family or group therapies. Our job is to help the client and, within the bounds of safety, ethics, and decency, we do what it takes to accomplish this task.

9. Family Therapies

In recent years a group of methods has evolved for treating a family. The size of the family group ranges from husband and wife to a whole network of relatives. The therapy orientations have a similar wide range of approaches, extending from psychodynamic methods for separate members to methods for altering a family structure.

Chapter Topics

9:1. Some Concepts of Family Therapy

In its early years family therapy relied on psychoanalytic concepts. Often a family therapy session consisted of a sequence of short insight therapy sessions, in which the therapist began with one family member and then turned to another family member. During such sessions, the other members sat by and observed. But family therapy has increasingly developed nonpsychoanalytic approaches that focus instead on relationships in the family. Discussion of two of the concepts that underlie these methods follows.

Interactional and Relational Concepts

In an interactional view, family difficulties are considered to be a result of the way the members *interact or communicate with each other*. Examples would be parents' having difficulty in their sexual relationship, in reaching agreement over child-rearing practices, or in hearing and understanding each other. Perhaps there is a stalemate in the family in which each member has taken the position, "I will do things for you only *if and when* you do them for me." In this standoff, each waits for the others to provide services and care. No one initiates any move towards the other and interaction as we commonly think of it remains at a minimum. When we approach a family problem on this basis, relationship patterns, rather than one person's neurosis, are seen as the cause of the family problem.

A similar view of problems in family relationships derives from Bateson's idea of "complementarity." Each family member's behavior aggravates the unfavorable behaviors of the others. For instance, one member may be more authoritarian and responsible than the others. The other members become more passive and irresponsible; their lack of responsibility, in turn, makes the responsible one more active and aggressive. Vicious cycles result. The implications of this idea for therapy are far-reaching: *If a therapist attributes the problem to the escalation of opposite behaviors, the treatment focuses on balancing the family roles.* All family members should learn to share in the responsibility for changing the situation.

The Concept That One Member Reflects a Family Problem

Many family therapists argue that one family member acts out or lives out a problem hidden in family communication or family relations. This family member is called the identified patient. For example, some family member remains psychotic or infantile *in order to prevent* change from occurring in the family. It may be that a couple has a very unsatisfactory marriage and both of them think they should get a divorce. They are unable to take this step, however, because each fears being alone. They remain married and claim that they stay together because one of their children has "problems." The child obliges and bears the symptoms in order to protect family cohesion.

9:2. Indications and Arrangements

Some therapists argue that family therapy is indicated only when the members of a family have obvious difficulties with each other, especially if the family members must or intend to remain together. But many family therapists have a broader view of the indications for family therapy. They do family therapy, although only one person may exhibit symptoms or difficulties, claiming that any symptom is a reflection of underlying difficulties in the entire family unit. There are those family therapists who take the position that family therapy is appropriate even for a client who lives alone. They contend that the client must be seen with other family members, so that they will make attempts to bring separated members together at the sessions, even though only one of them has the complaints. *The indications for family therapy, then, depend on our point of view.*

Usually all members of a household constitute the unit of treatment. Often this unit consists of one or two parents and their small children. Occasionally, it includes grandparents, other relatives, boarders, or the fiancé of a separated parent. Those therapists who insist on including all relevant family members in the therapy will not see various members separately. Some will not continue the therapy if all members do not attend. In practice, however, most therapists do omit small children from sessions and carry on the therapy sessions with whoever attends.

A treatment session generally consists of a therapist, one or two parents and at least some of the older children. Sometimes a co-therapist is present, especially in families with schizophrenic problems or in institutional uses of family therapy. Sessions are held on the average of once a week. A course of family therapy can last for several years, but short-term, time-limited versions are also used.

9:3. Doing Family Therapy

Imagine sitting with several family members. We will take the position that the immediate problem lies in the relationships among them and is not in one of them, nor is one of them the cause of the problem. On this basis, we proceed in a different manner than we do in a one-to-one session with a single client. We may use such familiar techniques as fostering insight, persuasion, support, suggestions, and the like, but we put them together differently.

Conducting the Session

It is customary to first introduce oneself to each family member, learn their names, and find out how each is related to the others. Then it is usual to get a picture of the problem. Most family therapists accomplish this task by going around the circle, asking each member to tell his version of the family problem. Often mother starts the account; sometimes father does. Some therapists concentrate first on the identified patient, that is, the one member with the most symptoms or the official diagnosis.

It is not always easy to get each member to participate. Some are reluctant to voice their opinions or even to speak at all. Sometimes one family member keeps interrupting or two members keep arguing about their parts in the account. The family therapist must interrupt them and use her best artistry to insure that each member is given a chance. The purpose is to maintain the initial task of gaining a picture of the family and the opinions of each member on the problem. It may be necessary even in these early minutes to make a confrontation: "You seem to argue so much that no one can ever make a point." Or, "Mr. Jones, you seem to do the talking for everyone in the family."

After the therapist has ascertained a preliminary view of family roles and behavior, he may be less directive and allow the clients to discuss or argue about the situation among themselves. *This allows us to see how the famliy members relate—that is, at least how they relate in front of an outsider.* But we also want to keep the dialogue flowing and preserve the therapeutic alliance. It may mean that we have to act as a moderator. We prevent family members from interrupting a quiet member. We encourage two family members to talk to each other, since they never do at home. Sometimes we have to prevent excessively violent quarrels or recriminations.

To facilitate open discussion we may find that we will have to resort to classical one-to-one techniques. We interpret why a particular parent is unwilling to allow certain issues to be discussed or we confront a family member with his tendency to blame everyone else. We can interpret defenses, as well as encouraging and reassuring members as we do in traditional insight therapies. *However, the main focus is on the relationships. We try to get all family members to understand what problems they share and how they contribute to them.* "Do you both see how you nullify what the other says?" "When your wife talks you always look down and away from her and whenever you talk she starts thinking about her arguments. You do not hear each other."

In addition to being a moderator, the family therapist tries to foster awareness of the fact that the family members *do not know how to initiate and sustain a discussion of the problem.* They do not know how to work towards a solution. *This is the problem we tackle.*

At least two differences in conception, then, distinguish the family therapist from the insight-oriented individual therapist. The first is the sense of being in charge. One directs the flow of discourse and does not permit protracted "free associations." And the focus of the therapy can be on fostering more awareness of relationships and communication patterns, but not on insight in the psychodynamic sense, that is, not on increased awareness of personal motives.

A Course of Family Therapy

When family members have become able to discuss issues and listen to each other, deeper levels of understanding may begin to occur. The members can develop an awareness that they look at the same issue in very different ways. Maybe they can each acquire some respect for the different viewpoint. We try to help them. There are many life truths, not a single right one.

There are many other things family members can learn about their relationships. Perhaps each inflames the other and escalates an argument, rather than one or both being able to walk away from an argument or being able to reduce the tension. Maybe the parents have to learn that their policies of restrictions and punishment do not work with their children. They can learn to try encouragement and praise. Often parents do not understand that their relationship adversely affects the children and is reflected in their problems and symptoms.

These approaches feature an understanding of shared family problems and their accomplishment can involve a course of many months or years of family therapy. Consequently, some therapists try to speed up the process with more active techniques. Family members may be pushed to try different approaches and practice them. Sometimes family members role-play each other's customary parts in a family discussion. Some therapists use "sculpting procedures" in which the members adopt each other's postures and manners or group themselves in ways which more clearly illustrate how they relate and distance themselves. Some family therapists emphasize the scenarios that the family plays out, tracing the origins of these into the family history. A tactic here is to construct a "genogram," that is, a diagram of multigenerations of the family tree and their relationships. *Many tactics are used in the service of the overall strategy of changing the ways family members interrelate and organize their family existence.*

Some therapists also use a shortened course of family therapy which is oriented towards gaining improvement in one particular problem area rather than searching into the nature of family organization in general. For example, the entire course may concentrate only on a problem of sexual relations between the parents, on getting Billie to go to school, or on learning how to prevent violent family arguments. In addition, some short-term therapies help the family through a painful transition, such as an illness or divorce.

9:4. Two Newer, Short-term Approaches

In some short-term variants of family therapy, the therapist assumes an authoritarian posture and employs manipulative strategies in order to resolve the family's symptomatic problem.

Paradox Therapy

In paradox therapy, the therapist takes a family history, makes an appraisal of the family conflicts, and then orders the members to carry out steps that *seem to aggravate* the symptom or problem. When this technique works, the symptom or problem is reduced or alleviated.

A young teenage girl, for instance, refuses to eat and is virtually starving. This symptom appeared when her parents prevented her from seeing her boyfriend. The therapist ascertained that the parents' strong stand was based on a firmly entrenched sense of morality and parental responsibility. The therapist then ordered the parents to assist the girl in refraining from eating, since it is obviously more important for her to starve than it is for her to violate their sacred morals. The two positions, the daughter's and the parents', are reduced to absurdity. As a result, the daughter begins to eat.

In another example of the paradox method, a mother felt obliged to take her young son to the park every time he asked, since he would throw a temper tantrum and hold his breath if she refused. The therapist ordered her to take her son to the park every half-hour everyday for the entire day.

In simple terms, the paradox apparently works because it uncovers a hidden agenda or issue and then reduces it to absurdity. Within the framework of double-bind theory, we could say that the paradoxical approach forces the hidden contradictions into consciousness *and* then demands that choices be made on more reasonable grounds. The family in the first example was forced to choose between their daughter's attitudes and external relationships and their own moral standards. In the second example, the mother was forced to choose between her overprotective behavior towards her son and the impossibility of carrying out an assignment.

Structural Therapy

In simple versions of interactional theories, it is assumed that people cause each other's behavior. But we must notice that family members follow scenarios or programs in organizing their lives and their relationships. A family argument, for instance, usually follows a traditional script that is as repetitive and fixed in its outcome as the comedy routines of Abbott and Costello. Structural therapy aims at altering these ritualistic programs, usually by insisting on alternative ways for the family to proceed.

For example, a couple complains that their son sets fires by "playing with matches." Dr. Minuchin, a structural therapist, interviews the family and finds that the parents do not spend time with the child. The fires are started when they are out and when the boy is alone in the house. Minuchin orders the parents to spend time each day with the child teaching him acceptable ways to use matches. The therapist uses the task of teaching the child proper use of matches in order to teach the parents how to spend time with their child.

In another example, Minuchin conducts an interview with a mother and a teenage girl who is very large and very strong. The child refuses to stay seated during the interview and Minuchin reacts by stopping the mother's narration of the problem and insisting that she make the child sit down. The mother claims she is unable to control her daughter and avoids a confrontation of strength. Minuchin insists on their battling it out right then and there before they proceed with further discussions.

9:5. Some Differences in Family Therapy

There is little agreement among family therapists on which of the approaches is best. One difference that separates the more insight-centered approaches from paradoxical and structural ones, for instance, is the question of how authoritarian the therapist should be. Common differences also appear in the dimensions discussed below.

Degrees of Involvement

Dr. Murray Bowen recommends that the family therapist remain detached, avoiding emotional involvement with family members. He urges the therapist to act as a mediator or mentor and to encourage the family members to interact and work on solutions.

Dr. Carl Whitaker, in contrast, argues, at least in the case of the schizophrenic family, that the therapist must get deeply involved on an emotional and gut level. He recommends that the therapist struggle through deep attachments and involvements with the family members and yet try to maintain enough perspective to gradually lead the family out if its dependent, entrenched, and immature ways.

Doctrinal Foci and Pragmatic Approaches

There are those therapists who argue strongly for recognizing that the critical element in understanding a family's problem lies in some particular factor or reason. A variety of theories have been developed that illustrate this position: (a) Family problems are due to persistent and misplaced loyalties; (b) family problems are due to the members' fearing change; (c) family problems result from a lack of candid and honest discussions within the family; etc.

A therapist who holds to one of these positions will organize the therapy sessions around a discussion of the focal element that the therapist believes to be at the root of the problem. There are other therapists who prefer to remain nondoctrinal. They tend to deal with whatever current problems the family brings in for discussion. This pragmatic approach attempts to work with the immediate issues as a means of seeking ways to solve problems in general.

Differences about How Families "Should Be"

Within the family therapy movement, there are also differences of opinion about how family members should relate. Some hold that family members should always be open and honest with each other concerning all matters. Others suggest that there are matters that should remain private. Also, there are differences about what the parental roles should be. Some family therapists advocate traditional roles for mothers and wives, while others argue that the liberation of wives and mothers from traditional stereotypes is critical not only for personal maturation, but for family development as well.

9:6. Shortcomings of Most Family Therapies

We believe that family therapy has become increasingly more sophisticated in the last decade. But several concepts that bear on family relationships have yet to be generally understood.

1. It is critically important to gain a better knowledge of how families are organized in the *home or household*. What people talk about in an office and what happens at home are not necessarily the same. Many American families interact at home with minimal conversation. They do things, together and separately; they carry out tasks; they sit and do nothing—*and* they do not always talk about what they do or how they do it. Yet, therapy sessions focus almost entirely on what supposedly is said at home. There is little attention given to what people *do* and even less attention given to *how* they interact in various situations.

2. Family organization varies with social class, with ethnic background, and even with region and occupation. In most family theories, there is an imaginary normal or usual family—ordinarily one that is patterned after a so-called middle-class, mainstream American family. In fact, there are many kinds of normal and functional families that have little resemblance to the ideal models of academicians and many practitioners.

Thus, the family is a most complex subject that will not be comprehended by simplistic theories. But this criticism could be leveled at all therapies, for all tend to rest their methods and theories on simple abstract norms that form rather myopic theories from the richness of human experience. The best training for any therapist is a broad experience in the "real world," since few of the present notions provide us with the necessary breadth of viewpoint and know-how to tackle the problems of mental health. We take it as a rule of thumb that the more one holds to a doctrinal position, the more that is a crutch, stemming in part from the therapist's disconnecting himself from the "realities" and "complexities" of everyday living.

9:7. Not Getting Too Confused

Thus far we have described three quite different ways of looking at the problems of how family members or people in general behave:

1. The problem is in or of the client and is treated by focusing on the emotional, cognitive, or developmental influences within the client.
2. The problem is in the ways of interacting, relating, or communicating among family members and is treated by attending to relationships among those members.
3. The problem is in the scenarios or programs of activity in which each participant takes a part or a role and treatment consists of changing these programs.

It is easy to become confused about these views and many mental health workers are. These problems become very apparent when we first start to learn and do family therapy. They will also trouble us in group therapies, crisis intervention, and community mental health procedures.

An easy way to appreciate these concepts is take one and assume it is the real, deep, or true one. We can then ignore the others. We can practice that brand of therapy that will fit the one model we have adopted. But sometimes we cannot maintain this approach, unless we wish to be blind to the complexities before us. We will find ourselves faced with the need to use different modalities of therapy. Or perhaps we simply wish to expand our breadth by practicing additional methods. Consequently, we must master all of the concepts.

If we are to do this, *we must realize that one approach is not any more true or valid than the others.* Our behavior is a product of our inner and past experiences, our present relationships, *and* the traditional ways we have of doing and relating (that is, the series of programs we follow in our daily lives). In and of itself each part is inadequate. Each may be useful and practical, both as a guide in therapy and as a key to understanding behavior. Each may at times be useful for a therapist. Each may act as a useful focal point for a client to make sense of his life. Yet all parts become useful when we apply them to a more comprehensive understanding of the client and his problems. Even here, though, they do not represent real, ultimate, or complete truths in any abstract or scientific sense. They are simply ways of looking at behavior and of making sense of human actions.

10. Group Therapies and Social Movements

Group therapies also treat multiple clients simultaneously, but the group meetings are not restricted to members of the same family.

Early in the history of the group movement the emphasis was on individual psychodynamics in a group setting. Recent approaches in group treatments have focused more on understanding the interactions and relationships of the group members. Still more recently, group methods have used shared nonverbal activities rather than relying solely on language and dialogue. We are also witnessing the emergence of social movements that to some degree rely on group therapy ideas, though they are not group therapies in the usual sense of that word.

Chapter Topics

10:1. Indications and Group Structure
10:2. Classical Group Procedures
10:3. Personal and Group Experience Methods
10:4. Approaches Which Focus on Structure
10:5. Videotape Playback Techniques
10:6. Activity Groups
10:7. Permissiveness and Authoritarianism
10:8. Social Movements That Employ Group Meetings

10:1. Indications and Group Structure

People who are lonely, alienated, or socially unskilled are often referred for group therapies, since group therapy is considered to be a means of increasing their abilities to relate with others and enrich their social networks. Sometimes clients who have had a great deal of individual insight therapy are also encouraged to join therapy groups to increase their awareness of others and expose them to the problems of forming and holding social relationships.

Commonly, groups are composed of clients who are more or less peers in age, class, and cultural background, and who share similar problems. Groups of obese people, alcoholics, isolated elderly persons, psychotics, drug abusers, divorcées, and the like are often formed. Group therapy is also considered for economic reasons. Since multiple clients can be seen at the same time, there is a reduced need for a therapist's time. Theoretically, at least, fees for each client are reduced correspondingly. And, of course, many clients participate in group therapy because that is what the therapist believes in or prefers to do.

Most group therapists feel that about six to eight members is ideal in size, but often considerations of availability determine group size. Groups can range from three to ten or more in the more traditional group therapies. Some of the social movements that use the ideas of group therapy form groups of much larger size, sometimes filling whole auditoriums with "clients."

10:2. Classical Group Procedures

New clients in group therapy usually enter a therapy room and take seats in the circle of chairs that characterizes the arrangements of group therapy. Then some of the more aggressive clients may begin to talk about their problems, addressing what they say to the therapist. The group arrangement consists of a set of sequential one-to-one dialogues between the therapist and each member of the group. It is rather like a set of short one-to-one therapy sessions, in which each client takes a turn talking with the therapist while the others listen. Each client may talk about his problem and the therapist may make a confrontation or an interpretation. Then it is the next client's turn. The quieter clients will be encouraged to speak about their problems and other group members may ask them questions or offer comments.

More often therapists discourage the use of a format in which each client takes a turn speaking only to the therapist. Instead clients are encouraged to address each other. There are group therapists who sit outside the central circle and demand that the clients conduct the sessions. Usually they will refuse to answer clients' questions directly. In such approaches all clients are to be listeners, partners and even therapists for each other, while the official therapist mediates and moderates the process.

Often co-therapists conduct group sessions. A more senior therapist may recruit a less experienced co-therapist, who will be trained while working with the group. But the co-therapist can participate in a variety of other ways: She can gain rapport with some clients who do not warm to her colleague, as well as articulating alternative viewpoints and suggestions.

There is a popular group version of expression therapy: Members are encouraged to verbalize how they feel about each other. For instance, angry feelings are stated and expressions of rage and hostility are carried out in sessions. Members who learn how to do this are rewarded with praise or sometimes with mutual hugging. Similarly, group members may be rewarded for expressing how they feel about sexuality or for mentioning warm or positive feelings about each other. Primal scream techniques, too, are used in group settings.

These methods may foster insight into existing feelings and their expression, but they also employ conditioning and behavioral modification techniques, particularly in the ways the members of the group are rewarded.

10:3. Personal and Group Experience Methods

The traditional group procedures cover a range of orientations quite like those in family therapy. In the forms which allow each client to tell his problem to the therapist, insight is usually encouraged and each client should come to understand his particular problem. The other group members can learn something about themselves by being observers and they can support and encourage the client by asking questions or by supporting the therapist's position.

In the forms of group therapy which insist on direct interaction among the clients, the emphasis will usually center on the nature of relationships. The therapist will note the inevitable appearance of certain characteristic problems of social relationships: Ms. Jones ignores her peers and insists on relating only to the therapist as one might do a parent. Mr. Smith always gains the floor through sheer aggression, by having the worst crisis, or with some other trick. Sometimes two people develop a competitive relationship and use the sessions as a battleground where each attempts to win and defeat the other. Ms. Williams may try to be teacher's pet and tattle on the other group members, while Mr. White may quickly become a self-appointed therapist who tells everyone else what to do with their problems. Since these problems mirror what happens in most human groups, their development gives each client a chance to learn the nature of social problems and how to deal with them.

Group therapists argue over which of the two general approaches is better. Some advocate individual insight, while others claim that learning to deal with group problems is essential. Which approach is best largely depends on the client. Some clients have never had an experience with awareness procedures and need them. Others are preoccupied with self-searching and badly need an experience in relating to other people. We need not even get involved in the argument, however, since fostering insight and encouraging awareness of interactional processes are not mutually exclusive methods. Many group therapists use both techniques and a client can understand at the same moment both problems in relationships and his contribution to these problems.

There is another sense in which personal insight and the understanding of social processes are compatible. If the clients share a common problem they can learn how others feel about it and deal with it. In fact, *this is a major reason for convening a group, particularly groups consisting of people who have common problems.*

Group therapies of any type often are critical for socially isolated and lonely people: They have an opportunity to develop social ties within the group; consequently, it is hoped, they will also learn how to do so outside the sessions.

10:4. Approaches Which Focus on Structure

As in the case of family therapy there are also group methods that focus on the structure of the situation and on the programs or scenarios that people unwittingly follow.

An example is transactional analysis, which employs both psychodynamic and transactional theories. The transactional model holds that people get into difficulty because they unwittingly follow destructive game plans or scenarios. Transactional analysis is only sometimes used in a group setting, but when it is, emphasis is placed on the unfavorable scenarios that underlie the problems of the group and its members.

There are other methods of group therapy that direct attention to the formats which underlie relationships. The T-group movement holds the idea that groups develop in accordance with certain characteristic steps of group formation. Encounter groups often encourage members to learn how to assert themselves, but they also may focus on the ways in which confrontations are customarily played out. The methods of the Tavistock school manipulate and change the structure of situations so that group members can learn how group events usually occur. For example, the seating arrangements are changed or a group leader poses as a group member and acts in a provocative and angering manner.

In summary, there are three models in group therapy.

1. The simplest of these concentrates on individual psychodynamics within a group setting.

2. The interactional approaches stress how the members relate to each other.

3. The more recent approaches suggest that people behave and interact in accordance with traditional programs or scenarios.

10:5. Videotape Playback Techniques

One method of using videotape in group therapy is to tape a complete session and then play back portions at the next session. The recorded material provides the basis for discussion as the participants see and hear their previous interchanges. In another version, the therapist stops the video recording immediately after a particular event and then replays the segment. The group sees itself as it was just a few moments previously and can respond right then and there to the feedback information.

Group members are often stunned at seeing themselves and how they behave in particular scenes. We recall one example of a man who continuously complained of people unjustifiably accusing him of not listening to them during the session. Once he enjoyed the advantage of a playback where he and the others could observe his behavior. They noticed that whenever a member of the group addressed him, he looked down and away, as if not to attend to what they were saying. He argued that he did listen, but he agreed that his behavior gave the appearance of inattention and that this "turn off" could offend others. Even though he was listening, he acted as if he wasn't. *The playback provided the group with an example with which they could explore the importance of other behaviors besides just speech.*

One of the commonest means of learning group therapy is to become a co-therapist and work under the tutelage of a more experienced group therapist. Now that an increasing number of people are interested in videotape, the young therapist can also profit from the learning advantage of video playback. Watching oneself in action can be the best learning experience of all.

10:6. Activity Groups

The group therapies we have been describing rely heavily on discussion and a conscious verbal understanding of human experience. There are group therapies that focus attention on tasks of a more physical and artistic nature. Examples from artistic fields include art, music, dance, and movement therapies. There are also group activities that center on manual arts and crafts, physical games, and shared outdoor activities, such as camping, sports, and educational trips. In such therapies, the therapist also can make interpretations or the group members can discuss their participation. This serves to combine both verbal and nonverbal modes in an overall therapeutic process.

Activity therapies are variously explained as teaching skills, *or* assisting in the understanding of individual psychodynamics, *or* promoting social interaction, *or* fostering social affiliation and reducing alienation. In our view, *activity groups can accomplish all of these goals together. They do not do one of them and not the others.*

Recent forms of activity-centered, or "nonverbal," therapies encourage and teach clients to touch, make more adequate gaze contact, and move together in synchronous and cooperative ways. These approaches may appear in movement therapies or other activity programs.

In a special version called "forced hugging therapy," a therapist insists that autistic children and their mothers hold each other and learn to do so. These dyadic events usually occur in group sessions of multiple mother-child pairs.

10:7. Permissiveness and Authoritarianism

There is another difference in group methods that warrants our attention. Group therapies and therapists range along a spectrum from very permissive to very authoritarian.

In permissive versions each client is encouraged to bring up any point of view. Arguments are permitted, when and if they arise, but the members are not pressured in this direction. Clients are not forbidden to engage in personal relationships outside the sessions and any member can speak out. Such permissive versions of group therapy resemble the way insight therapy is conducted in one-to-one therapies.

Whatever the degree of permissiveness, the traditional group therapies also follow the general rule of insight therapists: *The "acting out" of feelings and emotions is discouraged and great stress is placed instead on talking about such issues.* Two group members, for example, might become involved in a private affair outside the group sessions. If this becomes known, the group members or therapists will insist that the affair be discussed in the session. The affair itself may be discouraged or perhaps encouraged, but it is essential that it be "talked out."

In more authoritarian group therapies the therapist may reserve the right to set the topic and do all of the interpreting or confronting. Or the therapist may insist on certain orientations, such as an emphasis on expressing anger. In some versions, a group leader may manipulate chair placements and other structural features of the group setting. In social movements like est the group leader even decides whether the member can leave the room to go to the toilet and controls the group by actively insulting the members.

10:8. Social Movements That Employ Group Meetings

During the Korean War it became evident that group sessions with American prisoners and Chinese group leaders were an important part of the Chinese "brainwashing" techniques. In these daily sessions the prisoners were to examine and confess their capitalistic ideologies and they were to learn the ideologies of their captors. Group members were praised and rewarded for describing ideas that complied with the Chinese communist doctrines and confessing relapses into their previous ways of life. These sessions did not resort to torture and they proved to be a very powerful means of group persuasion for some of the subjects.

In the last generation similar uses of group techniques have been made in America and Europe. Some contend that the adoption of certain ideologies is necessary for "mental health." Group sessions are used to get people to repudiate their existing ideas and adopt the new ones.

Group therapies of this type are probably not very different in principle from those traditional group therapies wherein the clients should achieve psychodynamic or interactional understandings. *But, in contrast with group therapies in the mental health field, these movements frankly employ ideologies that are religious, political, or social, and the group members ultimately gain membership in some national or quasi-national organization.* Examples might include the group sessions held by Protestant religious sects, women's liberation movement sessions, and elements of the "radical therapy movement" which foster environmentalist or new left political ideologies. In Europe similar procedures have been used by anti-psychiatry movements and radical labor organizations.

An influential movement of this type in contemporary America is est (Erhard Sensitivity Training). Groups of about 250 people meet in auditoriums for weekend-long sessions during which the participants are systematically deprecated and disallowed certain privileges. The leaders of est affirm that the movement has no ideological basis except possibly to emphasize an "Ann Rand" style of "enlightened" self-interest.

There can be no question that people who attend and join group sessions or conclaves in any of these movements are "helped," in one sense of the word. Many people feel better when they join a supportive group and accept a new ideology. The question that confronts us here is whether or not we accept "feeling better" as a sufficient outcome of therapy.

11. Using a Comprehensive Service Program

Some clients and groups of clients need more than a single therapist and a single modality of therapy. They may need psychotherapy, medications, and perhaps crisis intervention. In a modern comprehensive program, each of these services can be provided.

Chapter Topics

11:1. Crisis Intervention by Telephone

There are times when a crisis can be dealt with over the telephone.

1. *The mental health worker knows the problem and has a measure of rapport with the caller.* The worker will want to ask a series of questions to be certain the situation and the rapport have not changed significantly since the last contact. Before we can appraise today's call, we must bring ourselves up to date. "Do you feel like you did on Thursday?" "Do you feel worse?" "Are you taking your medicine?" "Did you try turning on the TV when you couldn't sleep?" Such questions not only provide the basis for knowing what the situation is like, but also serve to reestablish the relationship between therapist and client.

If there has been no change, then the reaffirmation of the mental health worker's involvement should become more obvious. "I think we can still work on this on Monday." "I'll stick by you." "You know I'm with you in this." Other comments can help restore the client's sense of perspective: "You remember, Joe, that you always exaggerate when you feel this way." "Mary, you always get depressed and think it is hopeless when your mother visits you." Also, there are practical reminders of an ongoing treatment plan: "Take your medicine." "Try to see how it is for the rest of the day. I'll be here all day and tomorrow should you need my help."

2. *The crisis and the action needed are obvious.* If it is apparent what must be done, the crisis worker can say so: "You have to get to a hospital." "Take the child's temperature and then call your pediatrician." "Can you get in here right away?"

There is no use offering advice if it cannot or will not be carried out. The conscientious worker follows through: "I'll call you around three." "Call me back this afternoon and let me know what happened." If there is any real doubt or if the situation appears to be worse, arrange an appointment very soon.

If the client is irresponsible, resistant to the idea, or too psychotic to follow through, any advice we might give will be insufficient. Other more direct action may be necessary.

Some advice is worthless: "Stay calm," "Don't worry," or "Stop feeling sorry for yourself" normally are phrases reflecting our own frustration or lack of commitment. With very few exceptions, such exhortations will not help the client or the situation.

11:2. Convening the Supports

The telephone call has come in and we have determined that a crisis does, in fact, exist. One of our first steps should be an attempt to convene the client's support network. In calling someone to help the client, we also call someone to help us.

While still on the telephone, we must find out who could be called. Is there a spouse, a parent, a close friend? Are there family members nearby, other relatives with whom the client has lost contact? Many clients live with their families, but some live alone. In either event we want to get as many members present as is possible on such a short notice. We can begin by urging the client to make the calls.

The client will hesitate. "Oh, he would never come." "I can't ask them." "I can't stand my mother." We must insist and persuade. "How do you know they won't come?" "Try calling them anyway."

In most crisis calls, we will not be talking with the so-called identified patient, but instead with an anxious relative, neighbor, or friend. The same urging and the same tactics should be employed.

If there is no one to be called or if the client leaves us with the impression that he will not summon relatives or friends, then we should suggest that someone else be called who can help until we get there: "What about your landlady?" "Is there an older woman you know in the building?"

Someone should get there, and if there is no one else to call, we will have to be that someone. If we can't, then we must see that the appropriate agency is notified and that action is taken on this crisis.

There are occasions when the family or social network can be convened and reasonably be expected to take care of the immediate problem. If so, the therapist need follow through with only a confirming phone call. But often the social support group cannot deal with the crisis. It will then be necessary for the crisis team to go there and meet with the people. In these instances, convening the social support acts as an interim measure by giving the participants something to do until the crisis team gets there. Moreover, the presence of a family or friendship network makes the crisis team's work a whole lot easier.

11:3. Going to the Crisis

The initial contact is usually by telephone. We make a preliminary assessment of the problem, attempt to do what we can by telephone, and then begin the process of routing the client through the mental health system. Emergencies require alternative action. *Crises require special mental health decisions. Today this often means going to the crisis.*

Within the community mental health movement, crisis resolution has taken a new path. The innovation of crisis intervention teams offers immediate assistance, since the mental health worker can say, "We'll be right there."

One of the important distinctions of crisis calls is that the *team goes to a crisis, not to an individual.* Team members complement each other, for they frequently deal with a family, or, at times, with even dangerous situations.

Ordinarily, the crisis team has critical backup supports. A psychiatrist remains on call in case hospital admission or psychotropic medication is necessary. Team members prepare themselves with the telephone numbers of relevant agencies, including the police, medical hospitals, and ambulance services. They must always be prepared for every event "just in case."

Despite the presence of backup services, the crisis is usually the field team's baby. The team members will continue the screening process, mediate quarrels, calm down the hysterical teenager or the suicidal father. In short, they will attempt to cool down the immediate situation. Like the worker handling the telephone call, they will need certain information and face certain initial decisions. They must decide if this is, in fact, a crisis or an emergency. They need, too, to determine who is in trouble and what the problem is, and to make sense of the setting. Yet, they have an advantage over the telephone interviewer: They can observe the setting, actually picture the relationships of the participants, and engage the people in a face-to-face dialogue. They have the here-and-now crisis right in front of them and they can deal with it as they think appropriate.

11:4. Cooling the Scene

A critic once said that crisis intervention is nothing more than applying a Band-Aid. This is sometimes true, but it is just as true that the crisis call often represents the strongest patch in a total patchwork effort. If nothing more, crisis intervention establishes the fact that mental health workers are on call at any time and are ready to lend a hand.

During the crisis contact several key principles ought to guide the team members. They have begun this call because they accepted a plea for help at face value. They have a preliminary idea of the "who" and the "what." They accept the notion that *if these people are in crisis there has been a breakdown in their normal means of handling such situations.*

The cooling out process begins with a focus on the anxiety that prompted the initial contact. Following the greetings and introductions and after everyone is seated, a team member might begin with, "Mrs. Andretti, you made the telephone call, perhaps you would like to tell us why you called." Or, "Susan, it looks like your mother is very upset." *Taking steps to solve the immediate problem means taking steps to clarify that problem for everyone present.* As soon as the team thinks it is possible, the problem should be redefined and broadened: If Mrs. Andretti says her daughter's behavior is the problem, the team will work initially with this explanation, but eventually they will lead the issue to a broader problem, for instance, to the relationship between mother and daughter.

Staying with the immediate problem does not preclude gaining other kinds of information. Who lives in the household? Who is in volved in the situation? Who is not there who should be? The team will want to learn what precipitated the crisis. Is this problem acute or chronic? Here the picture will be broadened significantly if the team can tease out a time frame. How long has this particular episode been going on? Have there been similar episodes in the past?

If the problem is determined to be acute, we will want to know what triggered it and when it started. When this behavior occurs, what do the people usually do? Does everyone share the same view of the problem?

If the trouble is chronic, the "problem" is definitely something else. If Uncle George has been an alcoholic for ten years, then today's crisis is not Uncle George's behavior, no matter how strenuously the family insists that it is. The problem lies somewhere else and cooling the scene means getting to that hurt fast.

Obviously, much of time the team has to play the situation by ear. But we can offer the following as guides to keep in mind as we attempt to deal with the situation:

1. Ask ourselves repeatedly: Why is this a crisis? Why did they call today as opposed to some other time?

2. *Who* is hurting and what is the symptom? Determining who may require some probing. In many instances the so-called problem maker is not even aware a problem is present. The ones who hurt are the others and the symptoms are reflected in the fact they made the call.

3. From the very beginning moments, we should be looking for ways to calm down all the individuals involved and to help them gain another perspective of their situation.

11:5. Immediate and Remedial Action

Crisis intervention begins with certain assumptions. The first and foremost guiding principle is to stay with the immediate issue. Long-term therapy plans can wait until the present hurt has subsided. Secondly, the team should remain in charge of the situation at all times. Thirdly, when it appears that the immediate issue has subsided, the team will want to start remedial action right there. This may involve nothing more than arranging for the identified patient or the family to come into the clinic. It may also involve offering assistance to the family in the way of helping them obtain some service such as food stamps, medicine, medicare, and so on.

Mrs. Andretti called the crisis service because her daughter's behavior upset her. There was nothing more she seemed able to do. Her total resources were depleted. Mr. Andretti was out of town working for two months on a contract. Their daughter, Mary, has had episodes when she became quite delusional, but today she has alternated between screaming at her mother and sitting in her room staring off into space and refusing to talk. Mrs. Andretti has spoken to her husband on the telephone and they agree Mary should be hospitalized.

The crisis team is faced with a choice. Either they accept Mrs. Andretti's story and focus on the daughter's bizarre behavior *or* they shift the focus. Once the obvious anxiety has been alleviated and tempers calmed down, the crisis team can restate the problem. Instead of letting Mary's behavior consume their attention, the team members might try asking what is happening in this family at this time.

In discovering the time depth of the manifest problem and the symptoms of that problem, the team gains a foundation for shifting the focus. Perhaps the daughter's more bizarre behaviors accompanied her father's accepting the out-of-town construction contract. Perhaps the daughter acts out her symptoms only when she and mother are alone together for long periods of time.

Whatever the lead, the question must be what is happening in this family?

If the team sympathizes with Mrs. Andretti from the beginning, they would have at least two avenues by which to proceed. They might try arguing that what is going on right now actually has positive features in a larger system. Perhaps Mary's behavior serves to keep Mr. and Mrs. Andretti together by preventing them from focusing on their own problems. Or the team might try sympathizing with Mrs. Andretti, showing her that they understand how hard it is for her, especially now that she is alone. Hospitalization may seem like the only alternative for the moment, but in the long run it really is not an alternative.

However, we caution against sticking blindly by a technique. The object is to restate the problem, working the issue into a larger context so that the process of remedial problem-solving can begin. The choice of techniques obviously will be based on what is comfortable for the team, but, here again, the technique must be supported by a clear idea of what the team wants to accomplish in reaching crisis resolution.

Our sense of crisis resolution is to work at reframing the problem from an individual focus to a family focus. This task will be easier if the team has assembled as part of the crisis call as many involved family members as possible.

11:6. Medications in Schizophrenia

Usually the antipsychotic medications include three classes of phenothiazines:

1. the aliphatics, such as chlorpromazine (Thorazine);
2. the piperazines, such as fluphenazine (Prolixin) and trifluoperazine (Stelazine);
3. the piperidines, such as Mellaril.

The aliphatics have a more sedative effect and fewer extrapyramidal side effects, but chlorpromazine renders the patient prone to severe sunburn. All in this subgroup can cause a fall in blood pressure. The piperazines have less sedative action and are less hypotensive, but they have more parkinsonian side effects.

Other antipsychotic drugs include the butyrophenones, such as haloperidol (Haldol), the thioxanthenes, like Taractan and Navane, and the rauwolfia drugs, such as Reserpine.

The initial dose of chlorpromazine (Thorazine) for a patient who has not taken the drug before is often a trial amount of 100 mgm about three times a day. The doses for other antipsychotic medications can be pictured in relation to the chlorpromazine dosage. Thus, for Mellaril the equivalency would be on a 1:1 basis. But the doses of Stelazine and Prolixin are much smaller, being respectively 1/20th and 1/40th of chlorpromazine.

Ordinarily, the doses are increased slowly until the goals of the medication portion of the therapy plan are achieved. These include reduction in hyperactivity, lowered assaultiveness, and decreased withdrawal. Delusions and hallucinations may also improve, but memory, judgment, and insight may not. Commonly, hyperactivity and combativeness decrease in the first week, but six weeks may be required for a noticeable improvement in thought disorder.

Usually, the dose of Thorazine is 300-600 mgs per day. There is considerable debate whether patients should be kept on maintenance doses for a long time, or whether the antipsychotic medications should be stopped or markedly reduced after the psychosis ameliorates.

11:7. Antidepressant Medications

There are three classes of antidepressant medications:

1. the tricyclic derivatives that include imipramine (Tofranil) and amitriptyline (Elavil);
2. the MAO inhibitors such as Marplan and Parnate;
3. the stimulants, amphetamine (Benzedrine), dextroamphetamines (Dexedrine), and methylphenidate (Ritalin).

The stimulants can be addicting and can produce schizophrenic-like pictures.

Use of the tricyclic derivatives also requires great care. They must be given carefully to patients with glaucoma, cardiovascular disease, or latent schizophrenic symptoms. These drugs can also precipitate manic disturbances in depressed patients. Ordinarily, then, these drugs are prescribed to people with depressions, depressive phases of manic-depressive disorders, involutional depressions, or sometimes in schizoaffective depressions. They may not be very helpful alone in reactive or situational depressions. *Depressive patients sometimes attempt suicide during the early recovery period.*

The usual doses of Tofranil and Elavil are 150-300 mgms per day. A usual trial of these drugs is about four weeks. The depression does not lift rapidly and, consequently, placing a patient on an anti-depressant does not mean that we can relax our suicide vigilance. Elavil is often helpful when the patient suffers from severe insomnia.

The cyclic or manic-depressive states often respond to lithium carbonate (about 300 mgm three times a day). This drug has severe toxic possibilities, so all patients on lithium must have a weekly lithium blood level examination. This is easy to arrange in the hospital, but for the outpatient, lithium maintenance proves a problem that the clinical therapist must endlessly contend with, for often the patient simply does not bother to go to the laboratory.

11:8. Problems and Complications of Medications

Each of the drugs we have described has side effects. Some are serious and some are dramatic but not life-threatening. It is the psychiatrist's job to recognize and deal with these problems. It is also true that making diagnoses and prescribing medications fall within the legal jurisdiction of a psychiatrist or physician. But non-psychiatrists in mental health are often the ones who can first observe side effects or learn of complaints that require medical attention. Familiarity with medications and their problems, then, is part of the front-line worker's job.

The phenothiazines affect the basal ganglia and may produce two quite dramatic neurological pictures: The first of these is an involuntary movement of certain muscle groups, such as the neck or shoulders. Bodily parts may writhe and move in strange contortions. Phenothiazines may also produce parkinsonian effects. The patient experiences a marked decrease in mobility. It is difficult, for example, to move the arms or start walking. The muscles may also be rigid and a tremor may occur at rest.

This neurological syndrome is not serious and can be alleviated with additional drugs, such as cogentin and artane. *But* this syndrome must be distinguished from a picture called *tardive dyskinesia* which appears in patients who have taken phenothiazines for many months or years. In tardive dyskinesia, muscles of the tongue and face cause spontaneous movements. These movements indicate serious and sometimes irreversible damage.

There are other severe symptoms with the use of phenothiazines, including anemia, agranulocytosis, dermatitis, jaundice, and various metabolic and endocrine disorders.

The tricyclic derivatives produce side effects as well. These include anticholinergic responses of the autonomic nervous system, such as sweating, rapid heartbeat, low blood pressures and glaucoma. These drugs also produce blurred vision and dryness of the mouth, as do the phenothiazines. Also, sometimes they produce agitation, tremor, and other evidences of brain disturbance.

It is obvious what the mental health worker must do when these symptoms occur: An immediate consultation must be requested with a psychiatrist.

Insomnia is a serious problem for many schizophrenic, depressive, and anxious patients. Barbiturates and newer drugs such as Dalmane and Valium are helpful, but the barbiturates have serious side effects and all of these drugs are habit-forming. The problem of insomnia and drug dependence becomes a troublesome conflict for the mental health worker. On the one hand, the patient is quite miserable without help with insomnia; on the other, patients who take medication regularly become overly dependent on it.

Similar problems occur in the use of the highly popular Valium and

Librium, which are commonly given for anxiety during waking hours as well as for sleep. These drugs are habit-forming too, but they are prescribed almost routinely in many medical practices. A great many clients are accustomed to them and they continuously demand Valium or seek means of persuading the staff to prescribe the drug. Such drugs must be used with care. Rarely, if ever, should they be provided on an around-the-clock basis for long periods of time.

11:9. Comprehensive Clinic Programs

In the past clinics focused on one modality of treatment. Usually they were either psychoanalytic or psychopharmacological in orientation. Some still are, but many clinics today offer multiple modalities of therapy. This approach is well established in the community mental health centers that have appeared all over the United States.

There are several differences that distinguish the community mental health movement, at least in theory, from traditional programs.

1. The program is not necessarily headed by a psychiatrist and many of the key staff are "paraprofessionals" without advanced degrees in any of the traditional mental health specialties.
2. Multiple modalities of treatment are employed.
3. There is an emphasis on "resocializing" the client. In the place of the older idea of emphasizing differentiation and self-reliance, the community mental health movement stresses strengthening family and former social ties.
4. The emphasis is more likely to be on group activities, while individual insight therapy tends to be short-term.

5. Chronic schizophrenic clients are likely to be given medications as a major form of treatment, while other clients receive medications as a supportive measure in a more general program that is centered on activity therapies.

A desired goal is to enhance and develop a client's social affiliations. There will be an attempt to involve the client's family in the sessions or at least to increase the family's contact with the client. It is hoped that in the process family members will begin to assume more responsibility. More isolated and psychotic clients are brought into a "day hospital" where they have an opportunity to relate to each other. These relationships are encouraged by staff and are centered around certain shared activities, such as group recreation, games, dance therapy, and so forth.

Of course, it is for these very reasons that the community mental health center has come under rather constant criticism from established traditions. Unfortunately, community programs often fail to live up to their intent. Large numbers of clients may backlog on waiting lists and the client population may increase significantly without staff resources adequate for dealing with all of the clients. Crisis intervention workers sometimes end up bringing in even more clients instead of dealing with the crisis on the spot. Schizophrenic clients are loaded with high doses of medication without being actually enrolled in any other activity program and without adequate psychiatric supervision. Often individual psychotherapy in the program is inadequately integrated within the total therapeutic program of the center. It is inadequate in amount and quality in some clinics, while in others a few "choice" clients get endless pyschotherapy and others get none.

These problems in practice are often the result of immediate expediency, but they provide sufficient ammunition for critics to fire broadsides at community mental health. Lost in the process, of course, are the innovative ideas of multiple therapies tailored to the individual case and the humanism involved in helping poorer clients.

11:10. Modern Mental Hospital Programs

In theory, patients should be admitted to a mental hospital when they are dangerous to themselves or others or when they are too disorganized to care for themselves. In practice, other reasons often influence admission. Occasionally, the mental hospital is the only available, low-cost source of treatment. Sometimes the structured environment of the mental hospital is the only means of ameliorating an escalating cognitive disorganization. There may be more pernicious reasons as well. Perhaps a client's relatives wish to take a vacation and thus they dump the client into the hospital so that they are relieved temporarily of the responsibility of caring for that family member. Or it may be that the patient has 30 days of Blue Cross coverage and the hospital needs to fill its too many empty beds.

Whatever the kind of hospital and whatever the reasons for hospitalization, the incoming patient must face necessities of admission and confinement. Then in the final stages the patient reaches the point of discharge.

The Rites of Passage on Entering the Mental Hospital

There are state laws that make admission a legal step. Certain forms will have to be completed and certain procedures will have to be followed. These will vary with laws and institutional requirements. However, we might imagine the following as an example:

1. The patient may have to sign a voluntary paper of self-commitment or a relative and two physicians will have to sign a commitment paper if the patient is unwilling or incapable of signing.
2. A screening interview is held to determine the justification for admission and to gain an initial impression of the problem. During this interview a history will be taken and a psychiatric

assessment of the patent's mental status and preliminary diagnosis will be made in accordance with laws and policies.
3. Medications are usually prescribed, especially if the patient is diagnosed as psychotic.
4. Information concerning relatives, previous hospitalization, and insurance will be recorded.
5. The patient is sent to an assigned ward. During admission the person thus becomes a "patient" who must undergo further institutionalizing steps.
6. Most institutions and especially public mental hospitals maintain an ancient ritual that demands the patient be "deprivatized." He will be stripped of personal possessions, cleaned, and placed in a hospital gown.

These procedures have often been attacked for their lack of humanism, but, despite the criticism, we still have little idea of their impact on the new patient. We can say only that deprivatization is a step common in the rites of passage of many institutions, not only mental hospitals.

In the days following admission, the patient will experience additional steps in the hospitalization process. In the adequate mental hospital there will be an attempt to form a social bond between the patient and at least one staff member. Relatives may be included as well. A dossier of information about the patient's past life, a psychosocial history, will be compiled and placed in a file along with the records of previous hospitalizations and assessments of the patient's current life status and future prospects. The staff may also note in the first few days or weeks how the patient responds to various types of confinement activity and treatment.

This information is then used to draw up a treatment plan for the particular patient. In our judgment such a plan should include at least the following dimensions:

(a) a course of medication or a considered decision not to use medication;
(b) an individual psychotherapy or case management plan which allows the patient critical insights, personal discussions, and opportunities for planning and socialization;
(c) a program that includes group or family therapy, art, dance, or occupational therapy, and some ward milieu program;

(d) a plan for rehabilitation placement for post-hospital adaptation. This program of rehabilitation should begin early in the period of hospitalization rather than being postponed until the final days of confinement.

Such programs may be difficult to follow in many private hospitals, for each patient will have been in therapy with a private practitioner before hospitalization or will be provided a therapist at the time of hospitalization. Consequently, the private psychotherapy sessions will be continued during the course of hospitalization and the private therapist will make the decisions on what other program the patient should have. Some psychotherapists in this situation interdict any other therapeutic format on the grounds that their relationship with the patient might be diluted. We doubt that.

Many hospitals also employ a form of group therapy that is manifested as ward meetings of patients and staff. At these meetings, which may be convened two or three times a week, ward problems, social problems, and other issues will be discussed. An organization of patients may be formed with an elected chairperson, thus giving the ward a measure of patient government. These meetings, however, must be pictured in the wider context of generally encouraging patients to socialize. The ward, in effect, becomes a unit of focus, with these meetings and other group activities and parties becoming the means through which interaction can occur. This kind of program is often called a "therapeutic community program."

Finally, there is the matter of how long the patient is to remain in the hospital. Some patients are admitted for only a day or two as a means of carrying them over a crisis. They will then be picked up in an outpatient program. In the example of a psychotic break, the hospital stay may be a month or two. Some patients will remain for most of their lives.

It has been repeatedly demonstrated that a patient's readiness for discharge is not related to the severity of the symptoms. Instead, it is a function of the patient's life situation. Patients with very psychotic pictures can be discharged early to a supportive family and a tolerant neighborhood. In contrast, patients who prefer hospital life and have no relatives who care can become quite proficient at getting themselves readmitted. Hospitalization should work at avoiding any further erosion of family and friendship networks, since prolonged confinement tends to weaken ties to family and employment as it is. A good rule of thumb to remember is that chronicity breeds chronicity. Accordingly, we should be certain of our decisions whenever we recommend hospitalization or continued confinement.

11:11. The Three Legs of Contemporary Treatment

The idea of socialization or of maintaining and bolstering social ties represents an important new trend in mental health. It is quite different from the more traditional notion of fostering independence and autonomy that previously characterized the psychoanalytic era. But this trend also parallels a general trend in America today. There is a great interest in social affiliations and the old rugged individualism of the industrial era seems to be fading.

Socialization in mental health aims at improving the client's social connections and increasing the client's willingness and ability to form relationships with other people. It is reflected in the growth of group and family therapies, in activity programs, and in active efforts to bring friends and family members into at least some contact with programs of therapy. Further, the whole idea of community mental health has the goal of keeping the clients within their neighborhoods and not isolating them any further than they already are.

There is another trend, too. Prior to the introduction of the phenothiazines and antidepressants, most mental health workers were disillusioned with drug approaches and many were, and are, actively hostile to physical procedures, such as electric shock and psychosurgery. Previously, psychopharmacologists and psychodynamic therapists were opposed to each other. Few insight therapists would recommend or even allow medications to be given to their clients.

Now there is little question that phenothiazines are effective in ameliorating schizophrenic psychosis. Attitudes toward medications have softened and with psychotic clients many psychotherapists welcome or accept medication as, at least, a supportive help. Few therapists dedicate themselves to the exclusive use of prolonged insight therapies with schizophrenic clients.

Collectively, then, contemporary treatment, especially in the public sector, consists of some combination of individual psychotherapy or counseling, attempts at socialization, and medications, at least for psychotic clients.

These are the three legs of contemporary hospital and clinic programs:

1. *The client is to gain some insight and self-direction.*
2. *The client is to form and hold relationships.*
3. *The client is to have the neurophysiological equilibrium which can occur with medications.*

12. Using the Resources of the System

Using the resources of the system is simply putting the system to work for the benefit of the client. This can range from finding the therapist who works best with a particular client to "walking" a client through various community services. Any therapist must be aware of the available resources in a community, but this is especially critical for those who work in the modern comprehensive clinics. We will have to know how to get clients into various kinds of service agencies *and* out of them. At the same time, we must make ourselves aware of client rights and newer legislation that affect mental health so that the best care will be available.

145

12:1. Expanding the Range of Therapists

Working in a hospital or modern clinic exposes us to the interests and talents of immediate colleagues. We can take advantage of this situation by seeking advice or referring a difficult client to a colleague with special aptitude in dealing with the problem.

Even if we have a private practice we will get to know colleagues who can be called on to help with troubling situations. We cannot become familiar with all the therapists in our community, but we can make an effort to expand our network of professional contacts. These contacts can represent doctrinal differences such as Freudian, Rankian, family therapists, or behavioral modification therapists. Some of our contacts may have personal characteristics that will be useful. One may be authoritarian, another motherly, a third a maverick with anti-establishment ideas, and so on. The point is that we may be able to call on them because they work well with particular problems and particular clients. Some therapists will be excellent with depressive clients, others may be willing to tackle very psychotic or antisocial clients, and still others will be knowledgeable in psychosomatic problems.

12:2. Working with the Local System of Hospitals

Whatever we do or wherever we work in mental health, we cannot escape the need to make ourselves familiar with the hospital services that are available for client care. In many instances, we may turn to a hospital because we are as concerned with a client's physical health as with his mental health.

All hospitals do not provide the same services. Often they differ in quality of care and in accessibility of their services. Veterans hospitals, for instance, provide services only for some patients who have had military service. Private psychiatric hospitals accept patients only under certain conditions. Governmental hospitals are the most accessible, especially for poor and low-income people. They provide various kinds of services that range from city or county general hospitals to county and state psychiatric centers. A general medical hospital, whether private or governmental, often has a small psychiatric inpatient service.

As we become familiar with hospital services, we must learn the various intake criteria, eligibility criteria for use of services, fee rates, waiting periods, and the quality and type of care. Private hospitals, for instance, often differ in their psychiatric orientations. Some may specialize in only short-term therapy and multiple activity programs, while others may offer services limited to long-term individual therapy. State hospitals vary widely in the type of care, but they usually offer long-term hospitalization if necessary. A city or county hospital may limit the period of hospitalization.

General hospitals may or may not have a psychiatric unit, but they do provide other health care services. Most importantly, emergency rooms of general hospitals are open 24 hours a day, seven days a week. At times of emergency or crises and when other facilities are unavailable, a client can be referred to the emergncy clinic of a general hospital.

Special hospitals and hospitals with special services may exist in our community and the mental health worker will want to know about them. At our fingertips should be the telephone number of those units that specialize in acute toxic situations. Our list should also include special services for alcoholics, drug rehabilitation, medical convalescence, nursing homes extensions, and halfway houses.

The more we deal directly with hospital services, the more we need to extend our knowledge beyond simply familiarizing ourselves with available resources. The larger modern mental health clinics will probably have liaison people who deal with hospitals on a weekly basis; however, often we must be our own liaison. We must make contacts in the hospitals, making ourselves known to the various units and discovering those workers in the units who get things done for us. It is always easier to work with these institutions when we have a friend inside and one means of gaining and holding that friend is to provide some reciprocal service.

We recall the example of Mary, who was a conscientious psychiatric social worker employed at a state outpatient clinic. One of her duties involved liaison work with a local governmental psychiatric hospital. Her assignment included canvassing those patients who might be released into the outpatient program of her clinic or who might require long-term hospitalization at the state hospital. Mary took her work seriously and attempted to gain a picture of the staff and the hospital's care program. It didn't take her long to recognize that the intake physical examinations were routine and cursory. Moreover, she recognized that her social worker counterpart at the hospital showed little concern for her patients.

This knowledge proved valuable some months later when Mary had to weigh a report given to her by a patient against the statements of the social worker. The patient complained of being dizzy and reported that three years previously he had been involved in an automobile accident that subsequently had cost him his job. He had wandered aimlessly since, suffering, he said, from repeated headaches and dizzy spells. Mary wondered about possible brain damage and inquired if a neurological workup had been done on the patient. The social worker replied that Mary shouldn't pay much attention to the patient. He was a troublesome sort and a complainer. Besides, he had been given a physical examination during admission.

Fortunately for the patient, Mary was familiar with the hospital and was not the type to ignore a potential problem. She decided not to take a chance and decided not to push an argument at the hospital. She immediately began to arrange for the patient to be admitted to the state hospital. Mary had friends there and she could be certain that one of the first steps would include a neurological examination. There would be time enough to discover how troublesome the patient actually was.

12:3. Mustering Community Services

We may work in a clinic that provides a broad range of services. These services may be duplicated at other clinics and other clinics may offer services that ours doesn't. In order to provide the best possible care for clients, we should become familiar with other mental health agencies, making a point of learning their intake criteria, eligibility rules, fee rates, and special expertise or service programs that they have to offer.

There are a number of other human service agencies in our community besides those of mental health. We will find that providing services for our clients will also involve us in these other agencies. One set of service agencies we need to know about includes those that have special hot lines, such as suicide prevention centers, crisis intervention programs, the police, and the fire department.

Agencies like the Department of Social Services will prove particularly valuable to some of our clients. They can arrange housing as well as support supervised living arrangements. They can provide medical assistance payments and reimburse clients for transportation expenses necessary to receive medical care. They can help with homemaking services and the like. Other community services include job placement or employment departments, abortion clinics, family planning agencies, legal services, etc. The Office of Aging has various programs, such as nutrition programs, for the aged. Besides providing some services, the Office of Aging is also a primary advocate for the aged; any elderly client should be referred to it for assistance and participation in its programs. Offices of the State Education Department and local boards of education offer assistance by providing special educational help to many mentally disabled children and adolescents. The Office of Vocational Rehabilitation provides assistance in evaluating and training and often has a liaison with the state unemployment offices.

It is essential that we learn what and where these agencies are and how they can work for our clients. In many instances, providing the best care will involve much more than simply engaging in psychotherapy. If a client is to reach her optimal potential, the mental health worker will have to encourage her to take advantage of other human services and even sometimes guide her through the maze of governmental bureaucracies. Cities and counties often publish a community service directory and we should become familiar with that directory and have it available as a handy reference.

It may be that we work in a clinic that employs a social worker who specializes in guiding people through the various social service agencies. We will still want to have a general working picture of all these agencies, their organization, and how to deal with them.

If we do not have such a specialist available, it will be necessary to increase our knowledge of these agencies. We can personally get to know some of the caseworkers in these agencies, using them as our contacts and letting them teach us how the agency works. We can reciprocate by helping the agency caseworker learn about our services, by accepting referrals, and assisting on problem cases.

In working with other agencies, the mental health worker will have to share certain information. This may involve getting a client's informed consent if the information is confidential. It may also mean that as we work to help our client we will have to develop a plan in cooperation with other agencies. We should avoid duplication or contradictions, since most of the clients in mental health do not need the added burden of becoming involved in an impersonal bureaucratic process. Such a plan is essential because human service agencies frequently have goals that are not well defined and they sometimes unknowingly work at odds with each other rather than in concert. The mental health worker must be the person who stays on top of the situation, always working for the client's benefit.

In attempting to provide an adequate mental health care program, we may venture outside the formal government service agencies. We may have to muster other community srevices to help the client we are treating. We should gain an understanding of how our local community is organized and should have a sense of the community's flavor. Effective work in a community begins by identifying the sources of a community's strengths and its drawbacks. We learn who the leaders are so that we can call on them if necessary. Formal leaders are heads of political groups, social clubs, block organizations, and so on. Informal leaders are more difficult to identify, but as we work in a community we will talk with people and learn who plays an influential role in the neighborhood.

Many leaders are beholden to bureaucracies and organizations that tend to be self-perpetuating and do not necessarily hold the same directions as the residents of that community. In such a climate, the mental health worker must remain sensitive to the wishes and opinions of the different factions, educating them regarding our organization's goals and our product—health care. We should avoid taking sides or identifying our political beliefs or affiliations since this may lead to adverse reactions. It is hoped that we will gradually involve community members in some kind of collaboration and participation in our mental health agency—be it as volunteers, advisory groups, or even as members of a policy committee. We do not do this for simply altruistic reasons. Many governmental regulations, including those of federal and state governments, now demand an input from community members in the running of organizations such as community mental health centers.

12:4. Working in an Uncoordinated Service Environment

Mental health and support services have many sponsors. Some are sponsored by private citizen organizations or religious institutions. Some are sponsored by hospitals, both public and private, by medical schools and other educational institutions, by towns, cities, counties, and states. Further, in almost all instances, the federal government is involved either in joint financial sponsorship or in seeing that federal laws are upheld. For example, in New York City five medical schools, partly supported by government funds provide mental health care, jointly with and apart from city, county, state, and federal services.

The community mental health movement has extended the traditional range of mental health services. In rural America, community mental health centers are often under county administration, but funding comes largely from state and federal sources. The modern complex state mental hospital may have many branch offices and outpatient clinics with the inpatient hospital remaining as only one part of the complex.

This vast system of mental health services involves the worker directly in many units other than the clinic in which he works. At the same time, private organizations, volunteer agencies, special interest groups, community organizations, and the myriad number of other governmental social service agencies influence and relate to the day-to-day delivery of mental health care. Needless to say, the worker will frequently find himself working in an almost unmanageable service environment, with agencies duplicating services, contradicting each other, and defining similar and different goals for themselves. In some areas, there are efforts to develop unified systems of service among private, local, state, and federal facilities. If this happens, we will be able to readily draw on a broad array of services and resources.

Unfortunately, the integration of social services is more an idea than a fact in most areas. This means that the mental health worker has to tread through the maze, developing personal contacts, understanding the organizational structures, and making sense of the goals and priorities of other agencies. Since organizations tend to be impersonal and often indifferent, it is critical that we break through these barriers by making personal linkages and personal contacts with individuals working in the agencies. The exchange of interpersonal communication and the sharing of goals and work lead to a better understanding and act in the long run to provide direct benefits for our clients.

As we make these contacts, we must not only sell our product of mental health care, but also develop a listening attitude. We will have to bend our goals in situations that we might otherwise find intolerable and we will have to learn to appreciate that collaboration with other agencies means working within their operating system.

How do we establish such contacts? We pick up the telephone and call an agency, identifying who we are and why we are calling. We will also have to visit the agency, making it a point to talk with caseworkers about what they do and how they go about it. As in establishing any human relationship, we must make the effort and we must follow through. Eventually, we will find those people in the agency with whom we can work best.

Finally, any mental health worker who is employed in an agency will have to face the issues of the use of mental health manpower and the ways in which paraprofessionals and professionals are utilized. No matter what our particular methods or directions may be, we will soon have to recognize that we are influenced by factors other than simply therapeutic issues. Human service systems are increasingly being asked to show higher rates of productivity and to be accountable in terms of cost effectiveness. There are more and more regulations meant to assure high-level quality care which are mandated on organizations, especially by governments and third-party payers. In order to continually receive the various sources of financial support, organizations are asked to develop systems of evaluation through which the efforts and activities of that organization are measured by costs and results. Organizations are more frequently monitored by other agencies and asked to conduct peer review panels; their programs are continuously being modified so that effective mental health care can be provided in the most optimal and cost-efficient fashion.

12:5. Understanding Patient Rights

Practicing good mental health care involves more than simply selecting the appropriate therapy for a client or simply guiding him through social service agencies. It also includes protecting clients from the very mental health system that was developed to help them.

Clients have a right to the best mental health care we can offer. But any definition of the best will fall into a nebulous range of endless clichés. Standards of good care change. We once offered a blank façade and low involvement because we thought it best. Now many practitioners believe the best care is to become active and engage the client in the realities of forming relationships and dealing with problems. We used to promote an atmosphere of self-restraint, reduced aggressiveness, and sexual inhibition. Now we often encourage the opposite behaviors when we think it appropriate. *Perhaps, the best boils down to protecting our clients from sloppy care—and the best protection here lies in the personal morality, ethics, and sense of responsibility held by the individual mental health worker.*

Is there a quiet and arrogant sense of our professional superiority? Does it result in our dismissing opinions offered by clients and other nonprofessionals as invalid or naive? Has the term "client" become an impersonal reference that takes on the mechanical and occasionally derogatory meanings that hospital staffs often give to the term "patient"? Do we wittingly or unwittingly believe that women are more emotional, that Hispanic women are more hysterical, that Italians are more explosive, that Black-Americans are not responsible parents, that poor people abuse the welfare system? Israel Zwerling, Chief of Psychiatry at the Hahnemann Medical College, once said that the four enemies of good mental health were racism, classism, sexism, and professionalism. We could expand the notion of racism and include all forms of ethnic biases and prejudices. And we could include under professionalism the restraining and corrupting influences of doc-trinairism.

These are issues that we must resolve in ourselves and in our places of work. At a broader level, we must be aware of the civil rights of our clients and the increasing demands for appropriate care and treatment that are being made in the wider society. These demands, perhaps, are more pronounced for those clients who are confined within mental health institutions, and especially for those who are confined against their will. However, the concern for patient rights is spreading into the entire field of mental health and all of us are affected, regardless of where we work.

Most states now have a judicial review system for people who are confined in mental institutions against their will. Federal courts are becoming more active in these areas and are handing down decisions at every level which have far-reaching impact. For instance, in the so-called "Donaldson Case" the federal court decided that the state of Florida could not hold a person against his will unless adequate treatment was made available to that person. Similarly, a federal court recently handed down a decision against the District of Columbia, ruling that adequate community facilities, including residential sites, needed to be developed as alternatives to institutionalization in the treatment of the mentally disabled.

The mentally handicapped, together with the physically handicapped, are demanding rights of access to appropriate treatment sites, rights to education, and rights to employment. At the same time, various affirmative action groups are working towards reasonable employment opportunities for the mentally disabled.

It may seem at times that the practice of psychiatry is more highly regulated than any other health service. For example, in most states psychosurgery requires extensive review and approval mechanisms.

Similar efforts are underway to regulate the use of electroconvulsive treatment (ECT). These regulations and the complaints, however, may be justified. In the past, psychiatry and the mental health field in general operated free of many restraints. We don't have to read *One Flew Over the Cuckoo's Nest* to recognize the existence of snake pits, the violations of various rights, and the abuses inherent in the field.

Many responsive professionals argue that an appropriate balance must be struck between the need for immediate and effective treatment and the need to protect the rights of an individual. An individual should not be denied access to appropriate treatment, especially at a time when he does not understand the need for treatment. Overguarding his rights may result in more emotional or physical damage than might occur if immediate treatment were provided. It does seem clear, though, that physicians and psychiatrists, in particular, and all other mental health workers, in general, will have to give up sole authority over treatment decisions and subject themselves to the review of their peers and lay organizations.

12:6. New Legislation and Future Possibilities

In the early 1960s a Joint Commission on Mental Health released its final report entitled, *Action For Mental Health*. As requested by the President, Congress translated the recommendations of that report into a Community Mental Health Center Act. Federal funding was then provided for such services throughout the country. One also can expect that the 1978 report of the Commission on Mental Health established by President Carter will be followed by some congressional action and appropriation of funds.

The 1978 report recommends that gaps in mental health services be filled. Special attention was given to the chronically mentally ill, but recommendations were made for improving the care for children, adolescents, elderly, and those underserved in rural areas and urban ghettos. The most far-reaching aspects of the report have to do with the recommendations that an Office of Prevention be established in the National Institute of Mental Health and that within ten years some ten percent of the Institute's budget be allocated to prevention activities.

The commission's report marks only one set of recommendations for legislation. We can expect legislation changing commitment laws, thereby making it more difficult to deprive the mentally ill of their liberty. Such legislation will undoubtedly allow the mentally disabled the right to refuse treatment within a hospital setting. We can also expect legislation that will take cognizance of the District of Columbia court decision requiring the development of appropriate alternatives to hospitalization in mental health care.

In some states there is a clamor to involve mental health in the criminal justice system. An increase in mental health care in correctional facilities and prisons is therefore a strong possibility.

Whatever specifically happens in the Congress, legislatures, and courts over the next few years will undoubtedly create significant changes in the practice of mental health. Not only will mental health workers have to deal with a "patient's bill of rights," but they will find themselves working in an atmosphere that discourages authoritarianism and a strict application of the medical model, as well as a unilateral decision-making process in the delivery of mental health care. It is hoped that all this will lead to a better system of client care.

12:7. The Evolution of Case Management

There is a serious problem of discontinuity in the world of the mental hospital and the clinic. The patient may be admitted, discharged, and then readmitted again to the hospital. That same patient may be shunted from agency to clinic to hospital and back to an agency. Even while in the same hospital the patient may experience a number of changes—changes in programs and changes in personnel, especially when there are regular shifts of trainees who come and go with semesters or school years.

At some breaks in the overall discontinuity of health care, a new therapist may have to pick up from scratch and learn about the patient and about the patient's particular problems. Medical records and the patient's chart simply do not fill the gap here. At each break, the patient's sense of resignation and distrust may increase. Occasionally, he may feel that the only sense of continuity in an institution lies in the bricks and mortar that hold a building together.

The concept of case manager has evolved to provide a stronger sense of continuity. In theory each client will be assigned a therapist or case manager who will remain associated with the client for as long as possible, regardless of what other programs the client may enroll in. This relationship of client and "primary therapist" will continue whether the client is committed to a hospital, is assigned to a clinic, or remains at home.

Those institutions that are committed to the idea of case manager have had to create a mobile staff that can walk clients through the various steps the individual will take in the course of a broadly based therapeutic program. The case manager staff must be willing to make home visits, and become familiar with the various institutions, such as courts, police, county and state health agencies, that will form part of many client's lives. The case manager must also be capable of maintaining the relationship during readmission, even though this may place some stress on ward placement, ward practices, and the manager's home base clinic.

The case manager may be a psychotherapist and conduct a therapy program with the client. Or the case manager may refer the client to an appropriate therapist. In either event, the case manager must be willing to act continuously as primary therapist. Relatives and friends will have to be seen. The case manager may have to arrange her time so that she can attend group therapy sessions with the client. Also, the case manager must be willing, if necessary, to assist the client in such mundane matters as arranging a dental appointment or filling out an insurance form.

The concept of case manager involves some changes for the senior staff of an institution. They must be willing to designate authority for decisions to the case manager. They cannot expect a case manager to manage a case if the only authority yielded is to maintain records or to help the client get on welfare. For the concept to work, the manager must become the primary therapist and have control over the client's experience, whether this involves hospitalization or changes in the therapeutic program. Advice and consultations will be in order, but decision-making authority must also be delegated to the case manager.

12:8. Some Future Prospects

We do not believe there are sufficient grounds for continuing the old arguments about whether the psychological, social, or physiological aspects of a person's experience are more important or more "real." The trend towards integration appears to be developing and maturing. We expect that the need for case managers will become more obvious as time and events progress.

We can also expect to see additional developments in the three legs of client care. We can hope that psychotherapists will gain a better understanding of family organization and other network bonds, while at the same time evolving clearer and more effective psychodynamic concepts. Further, there is little doubt that safer and more efficient drugs will be developed too.

However, the mental health field will become increasingly more influenced by and responsive to national trends. Some of these trends will force changes upon the field, such that mental health will not be able to narrowly define its own purview. We see such influences already. Recent Supreme Court decisions require educational programs for institutionalized patients. Since patients now enjoy the legal right to an adequate mental health care, there are groups of people— both professionals within the field and people outside the field—who have taken up the crusade for client rights through various means that we can group as client advocacy. The results may eventually close the last of America's snake pits.

These trends and the corresponding changes in the approaches to mental health will also change training programs and clinical practices. It is not realistic to require nine years of education to qualify in medicine and three years of psychiatric residency to develop a professional capable of dispensing adequate mental health. It is equally unrealistic to require the clinically oriented psychologist-therapist to spend years writing a doctoral thesis that must conform to the designs developed in experimental psychology. And it will not be adequate to train all social workers as if they were going out to open a private practice in psychoanalysis or psychodynamically-oriented insight therapy. New kinds of specialists will be needed who can work with the innovations in the field, but who can also work with the traditional mental health specialists.

Mental health will need workers who are prepared for the newly complex field of mental health. A front-line worker must learn how to integrate levels of treatment and coordinate multiple simultaneous treatment programs. That worker will also have to appreciate the problems of inter-agency interface and know how to draw on the available resources in a community, whether they be the traditional helping agencies or voluntary agencies, clergy, attorneys, teachers, and neighborhood organizations.

III. Working in the Mental Health System

We do not do mental health in a vacuum. Instead, we do our work within a network of personal relationships, under various institutional arrangements, and according to a number of laws, ethics, and doctrines.

Occasionally, these contexts constrain and limit what we can do. Often they act as a guide and provide us with a foundation for doing our work. We must learn to work within these frameworks, not only for our own interests, but also for those of our clients.

13. Learning and Gaining Experience

Doing mental health requires a measure of formal education, specific training, and experience. Many issues, including career ladders, income, power and status mark the pathways to becoming an experienced mental health worker. As we gain training on the job, we also learn the value of working with others. Co-therapy relationships, supervisory relationships, and the intermingling of teams, groups, and staff meetings teach us a great deal about becoming an experienced mental health worker.

Chapter Topics

13:1. Where Do Mental Health Workers Come From?

Sooner or later someone is bound to say, "I guess you became a psychotherapist because you have so many problems of your own." The comment may come from a client, though more frequently it comes from our friends who are not in the mental health field. There is certainly a bit of truth in this old idea, but like all part-truths it is also a distortion. Everyone has emotional problems and "hang-ups" to various degrees. This hardly seems to be the issue, however. What apparently does characterize mental health workers is their opinion regarding how personal problems should best be handled.

There are many ways to deal with depression, unhappiness, chronic anxiety, or a tendency to foul up again and again. Some people seek their personal solutions by turning to the clergy, to alcohol, or to drugs, or by becoming perpetual medical patients. Still others withdraw and conceal their concerns, or blame others, or bemoan their bad luck. Then there are those people who think that the way to deal with a personal problem is to talk it over with someone else and to gain in the process a new slant on their problems. These are the people who tend to take up a mental health career.

A great many mental health workers have selected the field as a result of some association with the idea of mental health. Some have had personal or family experience with psychotherapy—perhaps a close relative had a serious psychotic problem or perhaps they had personal experiences with psychotherapy as a youngster or student. Others entered the field because certain courses at the university interested them and later the mental health field seemed to offer a challenging and financially rewarding career. Still others drifted into the field because they lacked a clear goal that would take them in another direction.

13:2. Formal Educational Programs

There are two general routes to becoming a mental health worker. The professional route requires formal education in nursing, medicine, psychology, or social work. The higher one wishes to advance in the career ladder, the more education will be required. Postgraduate work is necessary to advance as a clinical psychologist, psychiatric nurse, or psychiatric social worker. To become a psychiatrist, the student must plan on some five years of training and experience beyond the regular medical school requirements.

The other route involves on-the-job training. Usually, one's education and training will be in some vocation other than mental health. For whatever reasons, the choice is made to work in the field. For example, an artist may grow interested in art therapy, or a professional dancer might wish to study dance therapy and work in mental health. In recent years, an increasing number of people who lack a formal mental health training have been recruited into the field and then trained on the job to do mental health. They are usually known as paraprofessionals.

Professionals largely control the practice of mental health. Activity therapists and paraprofessionals are typically assigned ancillary tasks; if they do conduct therapy sessions, they do so under the supervision of a professional. But there are exceptions to this norm. In some public hospitals and clinics, nonprofessionals provide a much needed service, since regular professionals are in short supply. In these instances, few have time for supervision and some paraprofessionals eventually acquire an on-the-job competence that makes them excellent therapists —especially with clients from minority group backgrounds or clients who come from poorer families.

The Training of the Professional

Psychiatric training takes the longest to complete. A psychiatrist has two to four years of college, three years of medical school, an internship in medicine, plus three years of residency in psychiatry. It takes another two years of practice to qualify as a psychiatrist. Some psychiatrists take an additional period of psychoanalytic training that runs from five to seven years.

The clinical psychologist has the next longest training program. Ordinarily, it takes four years of undergraduate education, three to five years of graduate training, a year of clinical internship, and a written and defended doctoral thesis to qualify for the top positions in clinical psychology. Some psychologists also train in psychoanalysis.

The psychiatric social worker and the psychiatric nurse who wish to reach the top levels of their fields usually complete a four-year course of undergraduate training and then one to three years of specialized graduate training, thereby receiving a master's degree in their field.

Usually, psychiatrists command the largest incomes, as well as the most power and influence within the institutions of mental health. They do so because most mental health institutions fall under the aegis of the medical profession. Most hospital and clinic directors and many chiefs of service are psychiatric social workers. Research and training programs are often headed by psychologists. Nevertheless, the rule still holds and the influence of the medical model persists: Psychiatrists receive the higher salaries and occupy very influential positions within an organization's structure.

13:3. Institutional Apprenticeships

Mental health is a field that one learns in the doing. Although the professionals with the highest status have degrees, certificates, and diplomas that were gained after completing several years of formal education, the brutal fact is that these educational programs in and of themselves rarely train the student sufficiently in the practical aspects of doing mental health. Some have even raised an open concern about the merits of the formal educational programs in psychiatry, psychology, nursing, and social work.

Often the formal education is absurdly ill-suited for doing psychotherapy. A psychiatrist, for example, will spend some nine years learning to practice medicine and later will enter a psychotherapy practice in which the major portion, if not all, of that education will never be used. A psychologist will spend a similar period of time studying a wide variety of clinical and non-clinical subjects and then will write a thesis that is constrained by experimental theories and methods which will probably prove of little value later in the practice of psychotherapy. Many schools of social work feature training in psychoanalytic theory as if they were preparing their students for private psychoanalytic practices. Yet a large majority of social workers find work in the public sector where they will be working with clients and in situations for which psychoanalysis is inappropriate.

There is no question that these students gain something useful in their education, for they learn the theories and are exposed to the methods of the field. Most importantly, they learn how to organize their thoughts and tasks and they learn the value of responsibility. But only in the brief periods where they actually work as student-trainees in clinics or agencies do they gain a working understanding of mental health in action.

Often these first steps are abrupt. On day one the novitiate takes on cases in which he finds it difficult to apply the theories he has learned in the classroom. A great deal of anxiety can develop in those instances where he is not closely supervised. Sometimes this sink-or-swim method provides the student-therapist with an opportunity to mature quickly. In the positive sense, the young therapist will quickly learn how to work with people, how to use supervision, and how to disregard many of the academic theories that were offered in the classroom. But the danger lies in the other direction. The student can just as well grasp for crutches and evolve as a mental health worker who relies on simplistic doctrines and gimmicks that pass for tactics. With little else to go on, this trainee can easily become a devotee of anyone with an answer to his plea: "Tell me what to say to my clients."

13:4. Co-therapy Relationships as Learning Experiences

In many private practices, therapists work alone with their clients, but some practitioners form co-therapy relationships to treat families or groups. This is especially the case if schizophrenic patients are involved. Co-therapy is much more common in the modern clinics that feature group or family sessions.

Co-therapy relationships can take several forms. Often one therapist is a novitiate, the other more experienced. The more experienced member takes the lead in therapy and the less experienced tends to listen, learn, and say little. When the junior member does participate, he usually acts only to support the senior partner. This gives the impression in the sessions of the two therapists forming a united front, much as some parents do in relation to their children.

Unfortunately, these types of co therapy relationships have a tendency to develop quickly into dominant-submissive relationships, and the reasons are not always the result of competence or lack of experience. For example, the submissive member may be a woman, the dominant member a man, or the submissive therapist may be someone from a minority group background, the dominant member coming from mainstream middle-class America; or a psychiatrist may assume the dominant role and the non-psychiatrist partner may defer to him. The subordinate therapist may echo what the more dominant one *says*, thus maintaining the vocal façade of unity, while he displays facial expressions of disagreement or low involvement. Such relationships confuse and disturb clients, who readily pick up on the incongruities. *Co-therapists who find themselves in a dominant-submissive relationship must discuss and resolve the issue before they can engage in effective therapy.*

Co-therapists may take a united position for a variety of tactical reasons. Sometimes a course of action is so obvious that they agree a practical plan to achieve their goals. In this instance the united front becomes dominant, regardless of the relationship between the two therapists. A consensus of opinions held by both "authorities" also tends to carry a greater weight and to have a greater influence on the client than a single opinion. In other instances, a client may work away at dividing the therapists and they recognize the behaviors for what they are. They then may take a common stand and point out the client's uses of disunity as being adversive.

There are, of course, many situations in which the co-therapists do not agree. It may not be adversive or disruptive to allow clients to recognize that alternatives do exist. But the therapists should be on guard here. It is also possible for the therapists to take opposite but complementary positions. Each therapist, for instance, might deliberately speak to opposite aspects of a client's feelings and thus make ambivalences openly apparent. Another example might be for the therapists to represent opposite positions in a real-life dilemma and thus attempt to clarify it for the client and establish the first step in resolution.

Some co-therapists deliberately take complementary roles, with one therapist forming a close personal relationship with a client or family, while the other remains relatively detached, critical, and more "objective." One co-therapist may become markedly involved with the clients, sharing their fantasies and even supporting some of their unconventional actions. The other therapist holds back, so to speak, monitors the degree of involvement, and tries to maintain a broader picture of the course of the therapy. Since these tactics are highly controversial, inexperienced therapists might do well to wait until they have a bit more practical knowledge before trying them out.

Sometimes co-therapists simply do not agree at all and even develop a degree of mutual resentment and personal dislike. This is part of the politics of everyday living and, as in everyday living, there are times when it is necessary to either work out the differences or end the relationship. In therapy it is critical that these issues be confronted.

Co-therapy can be useful to all members of a therapy group. But one of its greatest values lies in the mutual support and learning experience that develops in the process of working with another human being. Discussions between sessions offer invaluable learning experiences and the opportunity to review a case with a partner.

13:5. Supervisory Relationships as Learning Experiences

Many institutions provide supervision for the young mental health worker. Sometimes these supervisory sessions are informal. They occur whenever the younger partner asks for them concerning a particular case. Sometimes they occur standing in a hallway or over the lunch table. But some sessions in many clinics are more formal. They are arranged at weekly intervals and the supervisor listens and comments as the young therapist goes over particular cases. Such sessions are an official part of the training in specialized therapies such as psychoanalysis.

Supervisory sessions ordinarily center on the assessment of the client and what the mental health worker can do. They also provide a more personal experience in therapy for the less experienced member. A supervisor may notice, for instance, that the young therapist makes consistent errors with client after client or that certain biases appear again and again in appraising clients. The supervisor can speak to these problems and discuss how they are related to the worker's attitudes, feelings, or perhaps even methodological fixations.

A supervisor may also take on the role of parent and attempt to guide the inexperienced trainee through the work of clinical practice. This kind of relationship can be most positive and rewarding, but it sometimes becomes filled with anger, domination-subordination tactics, and rebellion. Both supervisor and trainee must remain on top of their relationship, always recognizing why they are together and how they can improve their work together.

Some supervisors do not keep themselves informed of recent changes in therapeutic approaches. We find this to be particularly the case with the newer network type of therapies, which older, psychodynamically-oriented therapists may refuse to recognize. The less experienced therapist may be eager to try these methods out, but is discouraged or persuaded not to. A supervisory relationship should not become one of total domination. Sometimes paraprofessional workers who come from poor or minority group backgrounds resent supervisory sessions that become dominated by psychoanalytic models or models that more appropriately speak to the problems of middle-class America. Sometimes senior members in our field have had experience only with middle-class clients and they do not take into account ethnic differences or the actual life conditions of poor clients. An adversive supervisory relationship can also be a learning experience, to a point. But the paraprofessional and the young therapist should not remain locked in a relationship that is marked by continual restraint and criticism.

13:6. Teams, Discussion Groups, and Staff Meetings

In most contemporary clinics and hospitals, especially in community mental health centers, staff members are organized into working teams. Each team may have a more experienced social worker or psychologist, a consulting psychiatrist, and a number of paraprofessional workers, younger therapists, and students. These teams often have the time to discuss troublesome cases; students and inexperienced team members can find these moments to be valuable learning experiences.

Such informal discussions often take place over lunch, in the evening, or at social occasions. Mental health workers are notorious shop-talkers. These discussions are important for they help relieve tension, concern, and anxiety. Younger members of the team who may hesitate to ask for formal advice may inadvertently have their questions answered in the course of carrying on shoptalk over lunch.

Usually the members of working teams develop close personal relationships with each other and they may spend much of their work time and social life together. Discussions of clients and work may occupy their lives and come to endanger their relationships with others who are not interested in mental health. The young careerist can easily become seduced into believing that doing mental health is superior in dedication and human knowledge to any other life activity. This sort of chauvinism is unfortunate and we should guard against it. It doesn't enrich our lives if our friendship networks are reduced to only those people who work in mental health—reduced because others, including spouses, have grown tired of listening to us talk about nothing but clients and cases.

In some institutions the discussion of cases is formalized by weekly or monthly staff meetings during which troublesome clients and situations are presented and discussed. In private practice these work and discussion groups are likely to evolve informally, with young practitioners discussing work problems among themselves.

13:7. The Perpetuation of Ignorance

In the process of becoming an experienced mental health worker, most of us will overcome the shortcomings of our training and learn to deal with the anxieties of the early clinical experience.

But we face a new pitfall. We can become quite accomplished at mastering a particular doctrine and managing a single tactic. Some of us will grind out this approach, espousing its benefits, denying its drawbacks, and refusing to consider alternatives. We may do this for a professional lifetime. *The arrogance of past experience is really the arrogance of stultification, for we fail to learn from the present and we fail to explore for the future.*

In this sense, our clinical dealings become nothing more than making the same errors again and again. We can spot this arrogance when an experienced clinician leans back and calls attention to "my years of clinical experience . . ." Just as education and training can broaden or narrow our perspective, so can clinical experience.

14. Working in the Institutions of Mental Health

As we sit with a single client, a family, or a small group, our immediate focus centers on the therapy session. But the therapy is conducted within some institutional framework. The sessions themselves are part of the general activities of clinics and hospitals. These institutions also represent local parts of a larger system of mental health that includes city, county, state, and federal systems.

Organizations can become oppressive. They can hinder our work, but they also provide us with protection, opportunities, and supports. The more we understand the structure of mental health organizations, the easier it is for us to find ways to do our work as we wish.

Chapter Topics

14:1. The Modern Comprehensive Mental Hospital

The modern mental hospital is a far cry from the snake pits that were the picture of insane asylums of years gone by. Hospitals, however, still vary greatly in their appearance, in their ethos, and in the morale of the staff. Some remain largely custodial, while others feature multiple modalities of treatment, with the immediate goal being the imminent return of the patient to a life outside dependency and confinement. Some hospitals feature staff training and programs that provide the staff with opportunities to broaden their skills. Others offer few or no training programs and staff members get what education they can from other sources and in working with patients on a daily basis.

In seeking employment in a hospital we should look for certain qualities, since most personnel administrators are likely to claim they have a multi-modality hospital with plenty of educational opportunities.

1. We will want a setting in which we can work with a broad range of patients, some of whom *are not* chronic institutional cases.
2. We should note if there are regularly scheduled periods set aside for supervision, co-therapy sessions, and group discussions.
3. We should seek some impression of the quality of the senior staff members—can we learn from them and can we respect their work and opinions?
4. Are there informal and casual opportunities to spend time with colleagues?
5. Do physicians and psychiatrists dictate the course of events or is there a team atmosphere?

These and other considerations cannot be answered or learned in a single interview. The prospective employee must spend some time in the hospital, observing operations and meeting and talking with staff in a number of different settings. It makes no sense to rush into a decision. If the personnel interviewer balks at this type of approach, then we think caution is well advised.

Organizational Structure of the Hospital

Many of the headaches of job hunting and work activities can be alleviated if we have a general picture of mental health organizations and a specific knowledge of the particular organization where we are or will be employed. Organizations differ in their structure, but we can note who sets the policies, how decision-making is done, who carries out the responsibilities, who can change policy and procedure, etc.

Generally, organizations tend to be pyramidal in structure. When this is the case, there is a corresponding tendency to flatten that pyramid by involving many of the staff into what is known as participatory management process. The general policies and goals of an organization are usually set by the funding body, as occurs, for example, in a state psychiatric hospital where the State Department of Mental Hygiene establishes policies, but remains responsive to the governor and the state's legislature. The interpretation of laws and policies and their execution rest with either the director of a state hospital or, in some cases, with a group of people called a board. The director, however, remains answerable directly to the Department of Mental Hygiene.

The participatory management process continues on down the pyramid of the state hospital. Immediately under the director may be a deputy director of clinical matters and a deputy director of institutional administration. Operating on the same level may also be an office of citizen participation, an office of executive coordination, an office of professional affairs, an office of program evaluation, an associate director for quality of care, and an associate director for program services.

An administrative system acts to support clinical operations by providing administrative services from a business office, personnel office, and other divisions such as food services, laundry services, grounds maintenance, security, supplies, laboratory services, pharmaceutical services, etc. Under the associate director for quality of care, for example, we may find an office of medical records and statistics, an office of clinical research, and a program for quality assurance.

Under the deputy director of clinical matters, we find the programs and offices that immediately include the mental health worker. The flattening of the pyramid in this division may approximate the following example:

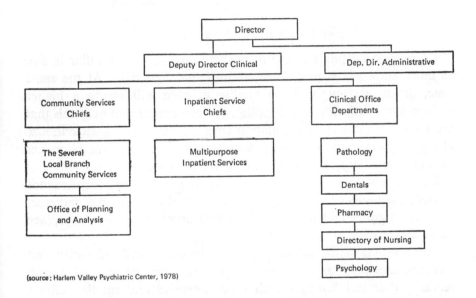

(source: Harlem Valley Psychiatric Center, 1978)

Budgets are prepared for both clinical programs and support services. It is mandatory in many programs that a system of evaluation be established. The mental health worker thus is part of and influenced by this information-gathering process. Data are collected, goals identified, and data analyzed in order to evaluate how well a program or division meets its goals in providing service for the number of people involved in the program, the kinds of people involved in the programs, the kinds of problems the people experience, and the outcome of these factors. While program evaluation is becoming part of the mental health worker's way of life, the techniques of evaluating are still not well refined and the outcome studies themselves do not well delineate what they are measuring.

When a mental health worker is employed in an institution, evaluations will be but one part of the paperwork that invades the work life. A system of documentation and maintaining medical records is another. Yet, here the keeping of medical records is designed for the benefit of the patient, since it provides for continuity of care, especially when a patient is treated by more than one person. The record also serves as a reference, offering the therapist concrete documentation of a patient's progress and of past programs and plans.

The Future of the Mental Hospital

Psychiatric hospitals of the future will definitely be smaller in size as more emphasis is placed on community-based care. At the same time, the newer emphasis on quality of care will assure a higher staff-patient ratio within the hospital. We can expect that hospitals that are far away from their population sites will gradually shrink in size and perhaps eventually be converted into other needed human services such as domiciliary care facilities or correctional facilities.

Hospitals will have to specialize more than at present, for demands to meet the needs of children, adolescents, and the aged will increase. Specific programs that relate to affective disorders may come to replace the focus on schizophrenia.

The hospital of the future will not exist as an isolated entity, but will become part of a comprehensive network of mental health services. Practical linkages with other agencies and satellite clinics will develop to service clients during the time of pre-care and of screening for hospitalization *and* during the aftercare programs. The "dumping" of patients on the streets should gradually become a thing of the past.

Finally, of course, the hospital of the future will become less the exclusive training site for psychiatrists and mental health professionals, for more of that training will occur in ambulatory settings like clinics and day hospitals.

14:2. Working in a Community Mental Health Clinic

With some exceptions we find two types of traditional clinics or outpatient services. One is the medications clinic in which the major portion of the client population will be dischargees from a mental hospital. These clients appear at regular periods to have their medications and life adjustments checked. The second type of clinic is the one-to-one psychotherapy clinic in which staff members hold a series of daily 50-minute sessions with individual clients on a short-term or long-term basis. Some of these clinics are psychoanalytic in orientation and do not offer a range of treatment modalities. However, more and more clinics now offer a broader range of services for mental health clients.

Clinics, too, are organizations and they can have all the disadvantages and advantages of the mental hospital. At one extreme are those clinics whose purpose seems to be getting in as many patient hours as possible. The availability of medicaid, city, county, state, and federal funds leads some clinics, then, to *sacrifice the quality of care for number of client hours.* At the other extreme are clinics that focus heavily on staff education. But education can also function at the expense of client care. Clients may be chosen precisely because they represent "good teaching cases."

In seeking employment in a clinic, we should look to a balance between a good standard of client care and education.

The Community Mental Health Clinic

The formal beginnings of the community mental health movement date to the 1960s and the implementation of the recommendations of the Joint Commission on Mental Health. The community mental health clinic differs from other outpatient services:

1. It is ordinarily community-based and governed, at least in theory, by the local community board.
2. It offers a broad spectrum of mental health and social services.
3. It accepts clients from all ethnic and social class backgrounds, from all categories of mental illnesses, and does not base acceptance on the ability to pay.
4. It is not necessarily administered by a psychiatrist and we are more likely to see many paraprofessionals and activity specialists working alongside and with professionals.

A community mental health center is funded through federal funds and the basic policies are those stemming from federal guidelines. Some flexibility appears in these otherwise rigid guidelines when a local board assumes operational responsibility for running the center. Obviously, the board must function within the federal and state frameworks, but the interpretation and execution of laws and policies rest with the board and director of a particular center.

This system of organization allows for great variability in community clinics and in some respect demonstrates why many clinics fail to realize their goals. Some clinics focus on long-term psychotherapy with a few selected clients while other clients go on waiting list. Other clinics seek an extreme form of cost-efficiency in which the number of services and number of clients become the goals. Sometimes clinics are ruled by a board of local citizens that is mainly concerned with using the clinic as a means of keeping "riffraff" under control. Some clinics are controlled by local boards whose primary interest is affirmative action and the advocacy of client rights. Staff may be undertrained or ill-trained in traditional therapies. Clinical settings may be utterly chaotic, with clients receiving very little in the way of what traditional psychotherapists would call therapy.

Despite these and other shortcomings, community mental health centers in general provide service opportunities for the clients and potentially exciting places to work for the staff. One can try out various therapies. In many clinics there is an organized program of multi-modality treatment. Staff tend to work in teams that are interdisciplinary, and education of the staff is an important ingredient. Most importantly, the community-based clinic offers the mental health worker the opportunity to learn something of the weaknesses and strengths of the neighborhoods from which the clients come and in which the center is based. There is a chance to work with clients from various ethnic backgrounds and social classes and to work with all types of problems.

The Organization of the Community Mental Health Center

Community clinics are often branch satellites of larger organizations at the county or state level. Each center is responsible for providing services in its district. Clinical executives, that is, people with clinical knowledge and management expertise, are frequently chosen to head community clinics, though the local board may maintain close control over operations.

Professionals and paraprofessionals are hired to perform particular functions and serve particular clients. Specific programs may include a walk-in clinic, day hospital, family therapy sessions, multi-group sessions, a social rehabilitation program, a program of regular home visits, a sheltered work activity program, and a 24-hour crisis intervention service. Whatever the program, it will usually be staffed by an interdisciplinary team. It is this team approach that characterizes a community mental health center. The composition of a team varies from program to program and depends on the particular functions of a program.

Just as the mental hospital is subject to reviews and evaluations, so is the community-based clinic. But the hospital is usually connected directly into a state system. A community facility, on the other hand, is subject to both local and federal guidelines. Funding is largely federal, flowing from the Department of Health, Education and Welfare which is the source of specific funds, such as medicare and other medical assistances. Federal organizations thus periodically review medical records, as does the Joint Commission for Accreditation. The latter agency not only reviews a facility, but also provides a certificate of accreditation that entitles the clinic to receive funds from other third-party payers.

The Future of Community Mental Health

The community mental health movement may have a shaky future. We are at a time when psychiatry is shifting more and more towards the medical model. It is primarily attempting to find its place as a discipline that can respond to mental illness through organic methods and chemotherapy. This trend is further facilitated by the clamor of mental health advocates to include mental health coverage in any emerging national health insurance. This could further narrow psychiatry into a medical definition of mental health and mental illness.

These directions might be destructive for the community mental health center concept as we know it as the present time. It might divert the necessary social and community mental health approaches away from the present mental health system and place them in the social services system. This, in some manner, might be desirable, because one of the major gaps in the present community mental health system is that it tends to remain isolated and not integrated with other human services. The report of the President's Commission, as well as the report of the General Accounting Office to the Congress, has indicated this need to integrate the mental health system with other human service agencies. Hence, the community mental health center activities in the future might fall within the purview of social rehabilitation activities sponsored by the Department of Social Services.

However, if some proven techniques of prevention of mental illness and promotion of mental health are developed, this may give further impetus to the community mental health movement. This could become a service specific to the mental health system and the mental health disciplines. If so, the maintenance and expansion of the community mental health system as a separate entity, but integrated with other human service agencies, may be the prospect for the future.

14:3. Using the Bureaucracy

Whether we work in a local clinic or a large mental hospital, our employment is part of a large bureaucratic system. For example, in a state system, the hospital and outpatient clinic are but two facilities in a network that makes up the large modern state hospital. But the state hospital is part of a system of administration that includes a hierarchy leading to the State Department of Mental Hygiene. And the Department is part of a state government in general that is controlled by a governor and legislature.

Various offices and agencies within this vast bureaucratic system function to see that mental health care is delivered. Payroll, personnel, and business offices are examples. To add to the bureaucracy has been the development of a civil service system which oversees the hiring, firing, promotion, and conduct of state employees. Since unions have also evolved to represent workers in these institutions, their contracts with state governments bind the state mental health worker to certain policies and levels of income. At the same time, the mental health worker is bound to certain principles and ethics, some of which are developed in professional societies. These various hierarchies of organizations intersect one another and often limit us in approaching mental health as we would wish. They also provide a measure of job security, sick pay, and health and retirement benefits, as well as guidelines for how we should comport ourselves in the system.

Some benefits result directly from being a working member in this system. But some accrue tangentially. There is no question but that the one area needing clearer definition is ongoing training and education. It is here that the system can help or hinder us in doing a job for our clients.

In order for a mental health worker to maintain and improve his skills, he must have the opportunities to continually educate himself. A worker employed on the front line of an industrial firm is there primarily to regulate and coordinate the operation of machines that produce a product. These tools were designed by specialists who are often far removed from the worker. In the field of mental health, however, it is the front-line worker who is primarily the specialist *and* the tool or machine that produces the results for other human beings. Therefore, it is necessary that we keep our skills sharp and technologically advanced in order to provide the maximum benefits for our clients.

Obviously, employees need to work in a secure and evolving environment in which they can see opportunities for further growth, promotions, and personal achievements. Appropriate training programs further this process. But we will expand our skills most effectively when we function in an atmosphere of participatory management and when we develop a milieu of humane understanding and a participatory treatment plan with our clients. In this sense, we "use" progressive bureaucratic organizations for personal development.

Employees organize themselves into unions as a means of having demands heard in large systems like state and federal governments. Through these unions employees have sought benefits, salary increases, training opportunities, and a means of achieving advancement. However, organized unions provide only one source of using the bureaucracy. They also can become dangerous in the sense that if our total attention is fixed on winning contractual battles, we may lose sight of our primary purpose of caring for people who need help. When we lose this perspective we may well suffer a public backlash of the kind that occurred in the community mental health movement in the early 1970s.

14:4. Possibilities of Private Practice

There are certain realities involved in developing a successful private practice. One must be reasonably confident about taking cases in the absence of close supervision. One must choose a location where there is access and a market for one's services. One must enjoy those qualities that inspire some warmth and respect from both clients and colleagues. It sometimes pays to develop a reputation for being especially willing and able to handle special and difficult cases, such as schizophrenics, or severe compulsives, or psychosomatic disorders.

There are certain advantages to private practice. The income can skyrocket with hard work, a good location, and a steady stream of referrals. One is relatively free from the endless paper work and politics of the hospital or clinic, as well as the constraints of reporting to, and being under the direction of, superiors. But there are disadvantages as well. We do not get paid when we are ill or on vacation. We accrue no automatic retirement benefits. And private practice can be very lonely. Most insidious of all is the tendency of the private practitioner to maintain little professional contact and to grow narrow in thinking and unwilling to consider alternative methods or ideas.

14:5. Making Use of Professional Societies

Meetings sometimes seem to form a major part of the mental health worker's life. There are any number of business and discussion meetings held within an institution. In private practice we take moments to get together with our colleagues. And there are many professional societies that have annual meetings, monthly meetings, regional meetings, and sometimes special interest meetings.

In mental health we find three types of professional societies. There are those that are dedicated to particular disciplines: psychology, psychiatry, nursing, occupational therapy, and so on. These societies hold meetings, publish journals, send out newsletters, and take in dues. Large national organizations like the American Psychiatric Association or the American Psychological Association also have regional, state, and local branches that act as subsocieties. These regional and local associations are part of the parent association, but they will carry out tasks that more directly fit the professional interests of their local membership. They, too, will hold meetings, print journals or newsletters, and collect dues.

The multidisciplinary society is a second type of professional organization in mental health. It is dedicated to issues that concern mental health in general and does not limit its interests or membership to one type of professional. The American Academy of Psychotherapy and the American Orthopsychiatric Society are two examples. The third type of society represents special modes of treatment, like the American Psychoanalytic Association or the American Family Therapy Association.

If one wants to maximize the advantages of these various societies, one probably should belong to at least one of each type. Being on a mailing list also keeps one informed of meetings and their agenda and publications. Those societies that are formed for particular disciplines or for particular modes of treatment are also known to guard the interests of their members in political, legal, and economic matters.

The cross-disciplinary societies are usually less conservative and regularly include experimental workshops and exploratory papers in the agenda of their programs and in their publications.

There are, of course, advantages in attending professional meetings. They can be educational. They provide a context where various ideas can be exchanged. They offer us the opportunity to see old friends and make new ones. And they have grown to become principal locations where people seek employment and employers seek applicants.

15. Explanation in Mental Health

The mental health worker functions within a confusing and conflicting world of explanations and doctrines. As we attempt to make ourselves familiar with the various conceptions of human behavior, we find our task made more difficult because some therapists and teachers advocate one approach over the others. This can range from a dogmatic stand denouncing other methods and praising one true theory to a steady reliance on a simplistic technique just because it seems to work in some instances. Throughout this handbook, we have frequently suggested that one theory or one technique cannot be adequate and it will represent no more "truth" than another theory. It may be useful to pause, step back, and look at an overview of what lies behind many of our concepts of the human experience.

Chapter Topics

15:1. Western Ideas of Real Truth

If we try to make intellectual sense of the doctrines that lie behind our field, we can face a problem more troubling than those brought by difficult clients. There are any number of theories and methods that purport to explain human behavior. There are biological views, several prominent versions of psychoanalysis and academic psychology, and various social theories of mental illness. On top of this are the people who treat a single approach as if it were the fundamental explanation of the universe. Of course, this follows from the general propensity in Western thinking to search for a single cause, a main cause, a fundamental element, or a real truth.

This tradition is not new, for we find a similar bias dating into the intellectual history of Greece. Since at least this period the Western scientific mind has sought to understand a thing by taking it apart. If this could not be done manually, it was done conceptually: The universe was broken down into component parts, a center was named, and then the parts were said to be held together by some prime mover. The individual has been treated in similar fashion and prime movers have ranged from vapors or humors to forces, instincts, drives, motives, emotions. The parts have been variously named, a most popular center being the psyche. This center in turn has been broken into component parts, as is done with the concepts of id, ego, and superego. All kinds of imaginary little people, or homunculi, have been postulated as living inside a human being.

This method of breaking things down seemed to work well in physics and biology and so the sciences of man tended to copy their more successful sister disciplines. Intellectually, this approach is now under attack, since there is pressure to put all these bits and pieces back together again. The trouble here is, however, that the imagined components are not conceptually comparable. The list includes physical components like genes, neurons, cells. It also includes the forces or actions, such as motives or instincts. It also includes the quality of actions, like masochistic or neurotic. But these lists are types of different logical orders. Since we can't put Humpty Dumpty together again, we spend the better part of our training learning all the different names and classifications of the separate pieces. And how do we use all this? We tend to pick out a favorite and say this is the critical piece that explains the whole. The problem is, of course, that another theorist can pick another piece. Again, we as students spend time mastering the various "schools" of human thought, but it is impossible to subscribe to all of these doctrines with their contradictory elements.

15:2. Explanations Influencing Mental Health

Like all organisms, humans behave. They do things. How we observe these deeds and how we put our observations together become our methods and theories.

The concepts of mental health have largely derived from scientific principles that are "thing-centered." Within this thing-centered orientation, we look at the object or the individual and the sickness is said to be "inside." Mental illness, for example, is said to originate in a person, gene, brain, mind, psyche. Recently, there are those who say the illness originates outside the individual, in the family or society, and *that* is the object that should be treated. Another version suggests we look not just as the individual, but at what the individual does to other individuals. This person does this and another person responds by doing that. There is action and reaction and we follow the ping-pong ball bouncing across the net: This is the cause, that is the effect; this is the need, that is the result.

Biological and psychological paradigms have mostly influenced mental health, but they, too, have been revised and changed over time. In the case of biological paradigms, the search for the cause of psychosis has shifted from diseases of the brain to disorders of neural transmission. More recently, the shift is towards seeing the disorders in the organization of neural processes. But most genetically-oriented theorists continue to attribute biological explanations to depression and schizophrenia, while claiming an experiential or "functional" origin for neurotic and behavioral disorders.

At the turn of the century, the psychological paradigm could be lumped into three major branches: 1. a holistic event centered, or gestalt version; 2. a psychoanalytic version; and 3. an experimental, behavioristic version. These, in turn, have altered over the years, leading to multiple Freudian and neo-Freudian versions of psychoanalytic thinking. Behavioristic models range through many academic subdivisions such as neobehavioristic and cognitive psychologies. The gestalt tradition evolved further in the 1930s with the field theories of Lewin. Currently, these views form an aspect of the humanistic psychologies.

To a lesser extent, sociological theories have influenced mental health. Interaction models have provided theoretical foundation for much of family and group therapies. Goffman, Szasz, and Laing have turned their attention to social processes and generally implicated society and its institutions in explaining pyschosis.

The Trend Away from the Trend

Other notions of human behavior have had a lesser impact on the field of mental health. The concept of evolution made it possible for us to shift away from organisms and things and to focus our attention on process. Einstein broadened our thinking by introducing a "field" view in which events could be described in time *and* space. This has led to recognizing that we can study behavior as a system of events and not something that emanates solely from the individual. General systems theory, cybernetics, neurochemistry, neurophysiology, and ecology are intellectual outgrowths of this way of thinking.

Early in this century gestalt theory and Lewin's field theory provided a direct means for mental health to shift away from a thing-centered way of thinking. Cultural views of mental illness soon developed, as did theories of conflicting communicational processes, of which double-bind theory is the most notable example.

But the problem in understanding and using these "event-centered" or process-oriented ideas lies directly in our training and in the biases of Western thinking. Most mental health workers find systems theory confusing and usually recast the ideas into a more familiar thing-centered universe. For example, today gestalt theory is often used simply to describe deviant cognitive images. The term "culture" is misinterpreted to mean a group of people: Black culture means all those Black folks rather than ways of behaving. Double-bind theory usually is reduced to those mean things parents can do to their children. Concepts such as "context" or ecology are thought to be other words for environment. In family therapy the family is often called a "system," but therapists see it at best as a group of people and at worst as an entity very much like the individual.

It is not easy to study deeds because we're too busy watching the organism.

15:3. Requiem for Conceptual Garbage

As we look over the field of mental health, we wonder if adequate theories predominantly guide our work. Certainly no one of the current ideas is sufficient, and certainly we have found no way to integrate the various ideas, precisely because they cannot be compared and integrated.

In everyday practice we often enter a session blinded by a particular doctrine that acts as a catchall for human deeds or we enter the session weighted down with several possible and conflicting interpretations of people's actions. The supposedly good theories that guide our thinking are rapidly reduced to "gimmicks," since we try to apply them with every client and with every case. The "good" theories we learned from our teachers frequently do not apply at all to the people we see in the sessions; when they do, it may be because we've lost the ability to see people for themselves.

We can practice therapy by trying out the various ideas. Or we can bury the whole mess. We'll offer this alternative, even though it may sound presumptuous and perhaps dangerous. Once we can rid ourselves of the intellectualisms of our age we might be able to see people as human beings again. Go to a session and simply listen and watch. Let the behaviors of the people sitting in that session do the teaching. Then describe the problem on the basis of what was seen and heard. Then work on a humanistic way of dealing with it and with them.

16. Keeping Well and Feeling Good

There are certainly no simple rules for gaining the good life. The experience of doing mental health does not guarantee our own well-being. Some mental health workers are happy and contented, while others are quite unhappy and sometimes unwell.

In our experience those who most enjoy their professions and lives apparently accomplish at least three things: They do good work, they make sense, and they maintain viable social networks.

Doing good work obviously requires a degree of responsibility and dedication. The rewards and recognitions of good work are more tangible for those who have acquired credentials. Maybe this is unfair, but it is the way of the established order. Another means of doing good work apparently involves making use of functional concepts, that is, a practical theory that guides the therapist in working with clients.

Making sense requires some degree of conformity, both within the general social order in which we live and within our work situation. This need not involve a slave-like obedience to any doctrine or life-style, for we need not believe blindly in what we do. Making sense means that we understand how to speak the language of our local world and that we understand the ticking of the clockwork around us.

Yet, making sense means more than simply knowing what to say. It also suggests that we solve some of our own persisting life conflicts.

Personal therapy may help us, but there is more to maturation than therapy. We can identify with some of our admired peers and seniors. And we can remind ourselves that we too have to learn how to form relationships and give our lives a personal sense of meaning.

One of the major problems in being a mental health worker is learning how to handle the problems that are built into the job itself. We are endlessly confronted with the inconsistencies of our responsibilities. We are to help clients, for instance, though we have insufficient time and resources to accomplish this task. We are to help our clients get out of the hospital and return for a try at living outside institutions, but local groups pressure us to keep them locked up.

There is no solution to these career problems, but we must endlessly deal with them while feeling a minimum of depression and cynical resignation. To do this we have to talk with our colleagues. There is no one-and-forever solution and so the process of feeling good requires an endless dialogue and a continuing set of social relationships, especially in our work.

We need a social network. We need colleagues who will listen, question, and comfort and we need colleagues so that we can reciprocate. Some mental health workers end up relating only to patients and clients as they get older. Some withdraw from their colleagues and professional organizations and relate only to members of their family. As a result, they become professionally isolated and often very reactionary.

It is also true that restricting one's network to colleagues can reduce us to insufferable professional bores. We need to experience the pleasures and problems of living outside a mental health framework.

A viable social network includes colleagues, family, *and* those friends who work and live outside the profession.

Bibliography

ANDREWS, M. "Poetry Programs in Mental Hospitals," *Perspectives in Psychiatric Care*, 1975, 13(1), 17-18.

BERGER, M. M. (Ed.). *Videotape Techniques in Psychiatric Training and Treatment, Revised Edition.* New York: Brunner/Mazel, 1978.

BOWEN, M. *Family Therapy in Clinical Practice.* New York: Jason Aronson, 1978.

BURTON, A. (Ed.). *What Makes Behavior Change Possible?* New York: Brunner/Mazel, 1976.

CANCRO, R. (Ed.). *Annual Review of the Schizophrenic Syndrome*, Vol. 5. New York: Brunner/Mazel, 1978.

CAPLAN, G. *Principles of Preventive Psychiatry.* New York: Basic Books, 1964.

CHAPMAN, M. "Movement Therapy in the Treatment of Suicidal Patients," *Perspectives in Psychiatric Care*, 1971, 9(3), 119-122.

CHODOFF, P. "The Case for Involuntary Hospitalization of the Mentally Ill," *American Journal of Psychiatry*, May, 1976, 133.

COLEMAN, D. M., and ZWERLING, I. "The Psychiatric Emergency Clinic: A Flexible Way of Meeting Community Mental Health Needs," *American Journal of Psychiatry*, 1959, 115(11), 980-984.

CONSOLE, W. A., SIMONS, R. C., and RUBENSTEIN, M. *The First Encounter: The Beginnings of Psychotherapy.* New York: Jason Aronson, 1977.

DILLON, A. "A Patient-Structured Relationship," *Perspectives in Psychiatric Care*, 1971, 9, 167.

DREIKURS, S. "Art Therapy for Psychiatric Patients," *Perspectives in Psychiatric Care*, 1969, 7(3), 102-103.

ENNIS, B. *Prisoners of Psychiatry*. New York: Avon, 1972.

FARHOOD, L. "Choosing a Partner for Co-Therapy," *Perspectives in Psychiatric Care*, 1975, 13(4), 177-179.

FREUD, A. *The Ego and the Mechanisms of Defense*. New York: International Universities Press, 1946.

GONZALEZ, N. "The Consumer Movement: Its Implications for Psychiatric Care," *Perspectives in Psychiatric Care*, 1976, 14, 186.

GRANT, R. L. and MALETZKY, B. M. "Application of the Weed System to Psychiatric Records," *Psychiatry in Medicine*, 1972, 3(2), 119-129.

HOLMES, T. and RAHE, R. "The Social Readjustment Scale." *Journal of Psychosomatic Research*, 1967, 2, 213.

KAPLAN, H. S. *The New Sex Therapy*. New York: Brunner/Mazel, 1973.

KING, G. "The Initial Interview: Basis for Assessment in Crisis Intervention," *Perspectives in Psychiatric Care*, 1971, 9, 247.

LAZARUS, A. A. (Ed.). *Clinical Behavior Therapy*. New York: Brunner/Mazel, 1972.

LEWIS, J. *To Be A Therapist*. New York: Brunner/Mazel, 1977.

LINDEMANN, E. *Beyond Grief: Selected Papers in Crisis Intervention*. New York: Jason Aronson, 1978.

LIPKIN, G. B. and COHEN, R. G. *Effective Approaches To Patient's Behavior*. New York: Springer, 1973.

LITMAN, R., FARBEROW, N., SCHNEIDMAN, E., HEILIG, S., and KRAMER, J. "Suicide Prevention Telephone Service," *Journal of American Medical Association*, 1965, 192(1), 22-25.

MACDONALD, J. M. "Homicidal Threats," *American Journal of Psychiatry*, 1967, 124(4), 475-482.

MACKINNON, R. A. and MICHELS, R. *The Psychiatric Interview in Clinical Practice*. Philadelphia: W. B. Saunders, 1971.

MARMOR, J. "Short-Term Dynamic Psychotherapy," *American Journal of Psychiatry*, Feb., 1979, 136, 149-155.

MAURIN, J. "Regressed Patients in Group Therapy," *Perspectives in Psychiatric Care*, 1970, 8(3), 131-135.

MINUCHIN, S. *Families and Family Therapy*. Cambridge: Harvard University Press, 1974.

MUECKE, M. "Videotape Recordings: A Tool for Psychiatric Clinical Supervision," *Perspectives in Psychiatric Care*, 1970, 8(5), 200-208.

NEHREN, J. and LARSON, M. "Supervised Supervision," *Perspectives in Psychiatric Care*, 1968, 6(1), 25-27.

NORRIS, C. "Psychiatric Crisis," *Perspectives in Psychiatric Care*, 1967, 5(1), 20-28.

OFFIR, C. W. "Field Report: Civil Rights and The Mentally Ill," *Psychology Today*, Oct., 1974.

OLIN, G. B. and HARRY, S. "Informed Consent in Voluntary Mental Hospital Admissions," *American Journal of Psychiatry*, Sept., 1975, 132.

PALAZZOLI, M. S., CECCHIN, G., PRATA, G., and BOSCOLO, L. *Paradox and Counterparadox*. New York: Jason Aronson, 1978.

PARAD, H. J. (Ed.). *Crisis Intervention: Selected Readings*. New York: Family Service Association of America, 1965.

ROBBINS, A., and SIBLEY, L. *Creative Art Therapy*. New York: Brunner/Mazel, 1976.

SAGER, C. J. and KAPLAN, H. S. (Eds.). *Progress in Group and Family Therapy*. New York: Brunner/Mazel, 1972.

SLOVENKO, R. *Psychiatry and Law*. Boston: Little, Brown, 1973.

SMITH, W. "Critical Life Events and Prevention Strategies in Mental Health," *Archives of General Psychiatry*, Aug., 1971, 103-109.

SMITH, L. C., HAWLEY, C. J., and GRANT, R. L. "Questions Frequently Asked About The Problem-Oriented Record in Psychiatry," *Hospital and Community Psychiatry*, 1974, 25, 17-22.

STONE, A. "The Right To Treatment," *American Journal of Psychiatry*, Nov., 1975, 132.

SZASZ, T. *Law, Liberty and Psychiatry*. New York: Macmillan, 1963.

TERMINI, M. and HAUSER, M. "The Process of the Supervisory Relationship," *Perspectives in Psychiatric Care*, 1973, 11(3), 121-126.

TICHY, M. K. *Health Care Teams*. New York: Praeger, 1974.

VAN HUBEN, B. "Exploration of Reciprocal Feelings," *Perspectives in Psychiatric Care*, 1964, 2(5), 43-46.

WHITAKER, C. "The Growing Edge of Techniques in Family Therapy," *Techniques of Family Therapy*. Haley, J. and Hoffman, L. (Eds.). New York: Basic Books, 1967.

WICK, J. et al. "Nurse-Patient Interview as a Learning Experience for the Nurse and Patient," *Perspectives in Psychiatric Care*, 1963, 1(4), 12-27.

ZINKER, J. *Creative Process in Gestalt Therapy*. New York: Brunner/Mazel, 1976.